A Doula's Journey:
Into the World of Birth

Sarah Goldstein

"This is a fascinating account of how and why the author became a labor companion for women and how she balances the needs of her family members and the women she serves." —Ina May Gaskin, midwife and author of *Spiritual Midwifery* and many other books

"An inspiring and gripping story of the many lives of a doula, told by one of the best. Sarah Goldstein, a leader among doulas, is a great story-teller who sweeps you into her complex and fascinating life as a doula, mother, wife and daughter." —Penny Simkin, author of *The Birth Partner: A Complete Guide for Dads, Doulas, and All Other Labor Companions*

"A deeply moving account of her life as doula, wife, mother, and daughter. Every page of Goldstein's memoir is steeped in experience, wisdom, and faith." —Henci Goer, Author of *Optimal Care in Childbirth: The Case for a Physiologic Approach,* the *Thinking Woman's Guide to a Better Birth,* and director of Childbirth-U.com

Copyright © 2014 Sarah Goldstein
All rights reserved.

ISBN: 978-1500889333

No part of this publication may be translated, reproduced, stored in a retrieval system, or transmitted in any form or by means, electronic, mechanical, photocopying, recording, or otherwise, without prior permission in writing from both the copyright holder and the publisher.

This book provides information and stories about alternate approaches to birth care. The book is for information purposes only, and it should not be used in place of personal care provided by a qualified physician or midwife. The author and publisher are not responsible for any adverse effects resulting from the use of information found in this book.

Some names have been changed to protect privacy.

Acknowledgements

I TRIED TO limit my questions, anxieties, over-enthusiasm and frustrations to a limited number of people because it is more fun sharing the finished triumphs. Therefore although they look few, the following people actually did more than the norm in assisting this book to be born.

Thank you G-d for giving me the strength and stamina to keep going.

Thank you to all the doctors, midwives, and long-time doulas who put up with me on the phone or in the delivery room. It took over 14 years for me to come to this point of learning and professionalism. After 6 doula courses, 4 conferences and various lectures, I have finally reached the point that I know I have much more to learn. I thank you all for your patience.

Mrs. Masha Fabian, Certified ASPO-Lamaze Childbirth Educator, who had confidence that my skills would get even sharper.

Henci Goer, author of *Optimal Care in Childbirth* for her long distance advice and guidance. Yeah for e-mail!

All the birthing women I have helped. Thank you for your confidence in my ability to bring out your physical and emotional strengths and allowing me to help you birth your babies with self-sacrifice (regardless that you may have chosen an epidural or needed a cesarean).

For their editorial services Gila Green, Chava Dumas, Shifra Devorah Witt, and Libi Astaire.

My sister, Alice, who supported me emotionally and helped as an organizer and proofreader.

My children who put up with days and many nights of the phones ringing, people at the door and your mom not always being there when you needed her. Thanks for your dedication to the cause of helping birthing women everywhere even when the "B" word became impossible to bear.

My husband, Moshe, who assisted with everything from picking up printing paper to how to word an idea. I hope one day he will catch up on those sleepless nights.

Table of Contents

Introduction 9
Chapter 1: A Passion and a Profession 11
Chapter 2: Mom and Dad 23
Chapter 3: Arriving in Israel 46
Chapter 4: Turning 42 & Facing Empty Nest Syndrome 53
Chapter 5: Finding My Path & The Course 57
Chapter 6: Mom's Diagnosis of Alzheimer's 65
Chapter 7: Meeting a Client 69
Chapter 8: Challenges in a Medical System 73
Chapter 9: Singing in the Rain & Moving Mom 86
Chapter 10: Why Women Become Doulas 98
Chapter 11: Choice, What Does It Really Mean? 107
Chapter 12: San Francisco & the Big Plunge 120
Chapter 13: An Interview with the Kids 126
Chapter 14: The World on My Shoulders, or Moving Mom to Israel 134
Chapter 15: The Wheelchair Birth 138
Chapter 16: Staff Relations & Finding Common Ground 142
Chapter 17: More Staff Relations 147
Chapter 18: The First Getaway 156
Chapter 19: The 16th Birth 163
Chapter 20: Blue Skies Turn Gray 168
Chapter 21: Doula-ing Spills over into Mothering 173
Chapter 22: The Bathtub Birth 186
Chapter 23: Spreading the Word 192
Chapter 24: Life Cycles 197
Chapter 25: Dancing with Mom 200

Chapter 26: Spreading the Word BIG Time   203
Chapter 27: Scissor-happy   207
Chapter 28: Hope Springs Eternal in a Doula's Heart   213
Chapter 29: The Second Getaway   218
Chapter 30: A Different Type of Doula-ing   221
Chapter 31: Personal Life/Professional Challenges   226
Chapter 32: Beyond the Call of Duty   231
Chapter 33: The Sandwich Generation   236
Chapter 34: The Induction that Wasn't   242
Chapter 35: Making Inroads & Staff Relations Improve   246
Chapter 36: Mentoring   254
Chapter 37: Mothering the Mother   265
Chapter 38: Car Crash at Midnight   270
Endnotes   276
About the Author   279

Introduction

THERE IS A major dichotomy taking place in Western society. As women are "liberated" from birth pains by choosing anesthesia and requesting major abdominal surgery called "cesarean," there is a large underground movement taking women back to the crux of birth.

For generations, women have been told that an episiotomy was helpful, that lying on the back for delivery was normal, that the baby didn't need her milk. "Bottle is Best" was the slogan. So my mom, like millions of others like her, dried up *my* milk, lay on her back and had the unnecessary episiotomy to help me come out.

We were and are continuing to be drugged because we are not "strong enough" to handle birth. We are given frightening scenarios and then told, "Why suffer when you don't have to?" The c-section is presented as a cure-all solution.

But with the right setting and support, couples *can* rise to the challenge of birth—and the doula (pronounced doo-la) is there to guide the couple as they make their transition into parenthood. She helps make the birthing experience understandable, normal and positive.

I wrote this book to give voice to the doula, to share my passion with future doulas and birthing moms. As a labor coach who is on call twenty-four hours a day, every day of the year, the doula is a woman who is often torn between her professional and her personal life. But it's my chosen profession, and despite the challenge of being in a sandwich generation—raising six children while caring for a mom with Alzheimer's—the excitement and satisfaction of helping women bring a new life into the world, plus my family's support, keep me going.

This is my story.

Chapter 1
A Passion and a Profession

DRAGGING MYSELF UP the last of the four flights of dimly-lit stairs in an old, stone building, I reach a familiar door. A beautiful olive wood nameplate greets me when I finally reach my client's home: Cohen.

Though Simon Cohen's phone call awakened me from a much-needed sleep, the combination of adrenalin coursing through my body and the climb have revived me. I am ready for action!

Knocking lightly on the door, Gail's six-foot tall husband cracks open the door and peers out at me with bloodshot, weary eyes. He looks weak and exhausted from another sleepless night.

"Thank you so much for coming," he whispers and welcomes me in.

"Where's Gail?" I quietly inquire.

"She's waiting for you," he answers, and points in the direction of the bedroom.

I know the layout of their small apartment. We have previously met for several pre-natal visits. An essential aspect of my job is to get to know the couple *before* the actual birth, so I can already be a familiar, comforting, informative and reassuring presence in their lives.

"How is she managing?" I continue, while we walk down the hallway together.

"We are getting tired," he says through a yawn. "Her contractions come and go and neither of us can sleep. Hope you had a nap after leaving us this afternoon. One of us needs to be rested."

When we reach the bedroom, I blanche at the stale air. I can barely breathe. "Hi Gail. I'm here. How are you feeling?"

She nods.

I ask her, "Can I please open a window?"

She nods again.

A fresh, revitalizing breeze rushes in. I inhale deeply and feel ready for the task ahead.

I turn my attention to the woman before me. Her eyes are closed, and she doesn't answer me as she stands and sways dramatically in a hoola-hoop motion. Rays of moonlight beam through the open window, silhouetting her full round belly as she dances rhythmically through the intensity of the contraction. She doesn't seem to fully acknowledge that I've entered her inner sanctuary. I wait patiently for the contraction to end.

"I need a drink," she finally responds, opening her eyes and lumbering to the side of her bed, where she attempts to ease herself comfortably onto a mountain of colorful pillows.

The water that I pour into the glass is the only sound in the still night, reminding me that during our last prenatal intake session, Gail had specifically asked me to bring a waterfall relaxation tape.

"Simon, can you get the CD player for me?"

Before he can answer, another contraction begins and Gail immediately lifts her heavy body back up and begins her rhythmic swaying motion again.

"Sarah... my back... the pain is so strong down towards the middle...,"

"Do you think you can try getting onto your hands and knees so I can massage where it hurts?" I offer. Gail gratefully complies with my suggestion and clambers onto the bed.

Kicking off my shoes, I get onto the bed behind Gail so I can get better leverage. I begin to press on different points of her back, asking where and how much pressure feels good to her. "How is this? Is this the right spot?"

"That's great—don't stop!"

I continue pressing through two more contractions, six minutes apart.

"I brought some aromatherapy samples with me," I mention for a change of pace. "The fragrances often facilitate a deeper relaxed state," I continue. "Here, try this." I sprinkle a few drops of sweet organic orange scent from a small blue bottle onto the back of my hand.

"Wow. That's *gorgeous*," Gail smiles.

I mix several drops into almond oil, and continue massaging her back.

My arm muscles always get a strenuous workout during long births. I'm making up for not having played tennis or lifting weights. Despite the winter weather outside, the apartment is warm and I need to peel off layers of clothing: first my cardigan, and then my vest. A cool, cotton blouse is enough. The beads of sweat are pouring down Gail's face.

"I am not sure I won't want the drugs."

"We said we will leave all options open. Right now you are doing amazing!"

I admire her for choosing this hard but rewarding approach. Witnessing the beauty of a woman whose body is surging with powerful hormonal energy gives me the momentum to continue. Each birth renews my respect, over and over, for the power of the birthing mother. It is sacred.

After three hours of position-changing, showering, applying back pressure and using relaxation imagery exercises between the now three-minute apart contractions, Gail wonders if they should go to the hospital. Though she preferred to have a midwife attend her at home, she is very conscious of the fact that Simon and her parents want her to give birth in the hospital. We had talked about this a lot during the two prenatal consultations. And now that we are in the actual moment itself, I see her wavering about what to do.

"My family is afraid of homebirth," she reminds me. "Anyway, I never even met a midwife." Simon agreed that they can leave to go to the hospital "towards the end." "Is that now?" They ask me.

"Do you feel fetal movements?"

"Yes."

"Your water seems to still be intact."

"Honey, we really should go," pleads Simon, whose anxiety wears away any semblance of the calm demeanor he had maintained for so long.

"No, please, Simon, I need more time here," Gail insists.

"Let's go well before the rush hour traffic begins, so

we don't get stuck on our way there," Simon continues.

By then, her contractions were two to three minutes apart and one minute long.

I decide to interject, "Gail, once we get there, we don't have to go in immediately if you don't want to. We can walk around outside, but at least we will be on the premises."

Gail agrees to this idea and we prepare to go.

The taxi ride takes twenty minutes. Rocking back and forth in the back seat, Gail moans her way through the bumpy journey, riding the waves of the contractions which are coming strong and frequently.

When we arrive at the parking lot in front of the building, Simon jumps out and starts unloading the suitcase.

Entering the building, Simon exclaims, "We had better go right upstairs!"

"No, not yet," Gail insists. "I need to find a bathroom first."

Knowing the hospital like my own home, I escort Gail quickly to the nearest bathroom just in time for her to vomit.

"This is normal. You could be in transition," I reassure her. "Do you want to stay here or go to the delivery room?" I ask.

"Soon, soon....Give me a couple of minutes. I don't want to hear that I am not so dilated," Gail explains.

When we emerge from the bathroom, Simon pleads again that they check in. Pressured by his nervousness, Gail agrees.

As we enter the reception room, Gail is relieved to be

welcomed by a smiling midwife. She is someone that I know!

Before she can lie down to be monitored, another contraction comes and Gail gyrates around the room.

"Please can you lie down now, so I can check you and the baby?" asks the midwife.

"I can't lie down, no way."

Turning to the midwife, I ask, "Is there a possibility you can monitor her while she is standing?"

"Yes, that's fine, but I can't check her like that."

I try to be a peace-maker/go-between for both—the staff and the birthing mom.

"Great heart tones," announces the midwife, reassuring Simon. The fetal monitor is removed, and Gail returns to her rhythmic movements that have helped her cope so well—squatting and hoola-hooping round and round.

Suddenly, Gail releases an intense scream.

The midwife checks her, announcing, "Wow! Wonderful! You're almost nine centimeters!"

"Just get the baby out!" she shouts.

We transfer into a private delivery room down the hall, Gail's fingers bearing tightly into my arm as she grasps me for support throughout the next surges.

I sense she needs me to direct her through transition. "Get in the shower! The hot water will feel great!" I tell her, while turning on the shower spray.

Twenty minutes later the midwife enters the room and insists that Gail come out and get monitored again.

"You need an IV, too!" she says, complying with normal protocol.

"Why do I need an IV? I don't want an IV. Am I dehydrated or something?"

"Okay, okay," answers the midwife, trying to be accommodating. "I do need to take a blood sample, and we can put in what's called a heparin lock— to keep the vein open."

"Pressure! I am really feeling pressure!" Gail shouts. She hasn't even gotten into a hospital gown yet.

Quickly drawing blood to send to the lab, the midwife then does an internal exam announcing, "You can push! I can see the head!"

Forty minutes of pushing and Gail delivers her 7 ½-pound, healthy, baby girl. We only arrived ninety minutes ago. With tears streaming down, Gail exclaims, "I'm a mom! I can't believe it! I'm a mom!"

After an hour of helping Gail to nurse her baby, giving her a hot drink and taking pictures of the new family, I make my way home just before dawn.

I quietly unlock our front door and slip into bed to get some essential sleep. The slits that are supposed to be my eyes are barely open. Much too soon, the sunlight streams through the slats in the wooden shutters letting me know a new day is dawning. It's 7:30 a.m. My children need to get on the school bus, something Moshe, my husband, normally takes care of on mornings like this. My arms, normally strong from kneading bread every week, are beyond sore. My leg muscles, still throbbing from squatting and supporting my client, slide off the bed, dragging all 5'2", 140 pounds of me to the bathroom. It has been another very long night. There is only one way to return me to a semi-functioning human being. An arnica bath followed by a deep muscle massage, were my only hopes for healing. Four more hours of sleep would be nice also. When will I quit this? Why do I go on?

I have returned from sweating through a marathon birth with a woman having her first baby. I was there for her, stroking her emotionally and physically for the endless hours of our time together. I am a *doula*. Some people are familiar with this term. Many have used our services. But there are still people who ask, "A doula? What's that?"

It is a calling, much more than a profession. It is a passion that we embrace: to go beyond our own physical and emotional limits to help a woman's transition into motherhood, encouraging her to access an inner strength that she does not even know she has. A doula is there to inspire. We cheer her on; "Just get through one more," or "You can do it."

I made a decision to help give women back the rite of passage. Now is the time to support women in making true choices based on knowledge from evidence-based medicine. Now is the time for me to help women have a positive, safe and rewarding birth experience.

Located in many countries around the world, this burgeoning profession was born from the birthing women's demand to have support during the birth process and the willingness of concerned women to be that special support person. Today's doula can be a woman with or without higher education. She can be of any age and background. She may have not even given birth herself. The main attributes she needs are a caring heart, a listening ear, strong hands, and a quick-thinking mind. She is a woman who has learned timeless comfort measures and techniques that have historically always benefited women.

The Bible describes the work of two Jewish midwives, Yoheved and Miriam, the mother and sister of Moses. They defied the ancient Pharaoh's cruel decree to murder the Hebrew slaves' baby boys. Courageously, they went about their individual tasks, Yoheved focusing on the actual delivery and Miriam comforting and cooing. Because of their pivotal roles, the Torah even assigns them second names: Shifra and Puah, emphasizing the importance of the work they were doing. Historically, birth was a woman-centered event, attended by capable, skilled, wise women. (The Talmudic word for midwife is *Hachama-- Wise Woman*). No woman was ever expected to birth alone, but rather with the supportive community of women to help her.

Throughout the ages, a woman gave birth in the comfort of her home, surrounded with familiar people. The midwife was a person the family knew well, her prenatal care provided in the privacy of the home. The other children participated in the welcoming of the new baby within their loving, secure environment, with no change after the happy event except for the inclusion of their new sibling. Relatives came to visit the family unit, helping with cooking, cleaning and sibling care. During their formative years, teenage girls bore witness to the miracle of birth; they knew it was a natural part of the rhythm and cycle of life. Mothers were not whisked away to a hospital for as long as fourteen days.

Siblings also understood without question that the normal, healthy way for a baby to receive nourishment was by breastfeeding.

Birth only entered the hospital setting in the early 1900's as doctors took over the role of primary caregivers. Doctors were the ones trained in medical interventions and knowledge of use of the "tools" needed to help women birth. A massive campaign evolved of the false "dangers of home birth", which helped convince women that hospitals were the ideal place to birth their babies.

Thus began the era when mothers were separated from their families, and mystery, secrecy and fearful trepidation of the unknown started to seep into the consciousness of young women. Now there was uncertainty in the picture: Where was mom? When will she return? If she is going to the hospital, does that mean she is ill?

A woman became vulnerable to the unknown variables of the hospital setting. She would no longer be in control of her birth, but rather she would be told how to move, when to use the bathroom, not to eat, and when and in what position to lie. Even today, a century later, (especially in America), there is little certainty that a woman will get her doctor of choice. Most practices embody a group of doctors, who assign the on-call doctor to the laboring woman.

A bit of history: In 1944, Dr. Grantly Dick-Read wrote *Childbirth without Fear*, based on his observations of European birthing women. He noted that fear contributed to pain in childbirth, and the goal was to educate women as much as possible so that they would not have fear of birth as a cause of unnecessary pain. Nine years later, Dr. Fernand Lamaze contributed his theory of how to facilitate painless birth, followed soon by Dr. Robert Bradley, who wrote *Husband Coached Childbirth* about the importance of the father's presence and support during the birthing process.

In 1956, the National Childbirth Trust (NCT) was established in England and in the 1960's in America, childbirth preparation classes came into vogue, thus giving a couple more knowledge of their birth options. The hospital staff, however, was still in control; insurance companies needed validation of practice in case of lawsuits; and the woman was as vulnerable to being subjected to unnecessary, and even harmful, interventions as she had been. (For example, "Twilight Sleep," the drug Scopolamin-Morphin was brought from Europe when American feminists chanted, "If European women have a drug to ease birth pains, then we deserve it too!" It was popular for over forty years. It seemingly removed pain but actually brought an amnesic condition in the woman removing all memory of pain and the birth itself. It was later discovered to cause respiratory depression and affected the infant's central nervous system. This resulted in a drowsy newborn with poor breathing capacity. Women were unable to push so episiotomy and forceps extractions were needed.)

Needing support, reassurance and advocacy, women longed for a non-medical assistant, someone who was there solely for the birthing couple, guiding them through the process.

"My husband is my left hand, my doula is my right." —A woman quoted in *Doulas Making a Difference*, a film by Penny Simkin.

"My doula was my anchor in a tumultuous sea of sensations. She was to me what a lighthouse is to a ship; a gentle guide steering me past hazards and leading me to my destination." —*Special Women*, a film by Polly Perez.

These statements transform my profession into a passion. It is worth being on call 24/7, when one is enraptured by the mystery, as well as the desire to serve.

I partially credit my own mother for my desire to save and protect the vulnerable of society, in this case the birthing woman.

Chapter 2
Mom and Dad

MY MOTHER WAS a short, thick-waisted woman, born in the Bronx, New York in 1927. The daughter of immigrants from Poland, she was born eight years after the last of three girls, and suffered during the poverty-stricken era of the Depression years. She wore large glasses that hid the kindness in her brown eyes. She was very self-conscious of the wide gap between her two front teeth, though my sisters and I assured her that she looked wonderful the way she was. She was our mom!

She used to tell us, often, in a sad kind of way, that her parents had three girls all close together in age, and then a long break of eight years before they discovered to their surprise that they were expecting a fourth child. They were very disappointed when she wasn't a boy. She seemed to have internalized their disappointment, which strongly undermined her sense of self-esteem. In an era when boys were considered the family bread winners of the future and girls superfluous, my mom grew up feeling like the fifth wheel.

Though her eldest sister went to art school, and her next two sisters attended college, my mom graduated high school at fifteen years old, finding a dead-end secretarial job. There was no potential for advancements or a lucrative career. She worked at this job for over seven years, before she met my father, a short, stocky man with a thick head of black hair, the son of Russian immigrants.

My father's own father had died when he was only eight years old. His eighteen-year-old brother, Sam, abandoned his widowed mother and little brother in hopes of finding fame and fortune playing the piano in any city but Brooklyn. His mother attempted to eke out a living, singing in local Brooklyn dinner clubs, while my father was left alone, wandering the streets, and often going to sleep in their empty, deserted apartment.

At the age of seventeen, he seized the opportunity to become an army "lifer", enlisting for a twenty-year service. This not only gave him the freedom of expense-paid travel and excitement, and an out from the poverty he grew up with, but a secure feeling of belonging, importance and self-worth. When we were children, he proudly showed us the photographs of his battalion that he kept in fancy leather albums.

When he was not abroad, but off-duty stationed at home, he enjoyed the USO (United Service Organization) social dances that were sponsored for soldiers. That's where he met my mom. He was a handsome, twenty-three-year-old young man in uniform, asking my mother, who was nearly twenty-four, for a date. After only three dates, he asked my mom to marry him.

Like most American families during the fifties, Dad was the traditional family bread winner, working as a soldier who rode on tanks, helicopters and had a variety of other duties which I was never clear about. Mom was the homemaker, working part-time in the morning, always there to greet us when we came home from school. When she did return to more full-time work, doing freelance market research jobs, it was after my younger sister Paula began elementary school.

Dad was an amazing story teller—creating a story around any character or object we randomly thought of. He asked us to mention a person or object and would weave a tale around them. *"A lollipop"*, my younger sister said. *"A dog!"* said my older sister. *"A little girl"* I chimed up and voila- a story! When he wasn't home to entertain us at bedtime, Mom would sing us popular songs by Doris Day and Barbra Streisand.

The army stationed my dad in different cities around the country and around the world. My older sister, Alice, was born in 1953 in an army base hospital in Fort Benning, Georgia. My mom doesn't remember a lot about the birth, only that it was a forceps delivery.

I was born eighteen months later, when they were stationed in Wilmington, North Carolina. One year later, my youngest sister, Paula, was born before our family relocated to California for a six-month stay. We were all bottle fed. Milk was dried up. Doctor knew best.

After California, Dad was stationed back and forth between Germany and Philadelphia for the next nine years. When we finally returned to Philly, I was twelve years old and anxious to settle into a "permanent" home and make long-term friendships.

When we were teenagers, my mother encouraged us to get involved in social causes. She emphasized that we were to help change things for the better. On Earth Day, April 22, I can still vividly remember how she rallied us to do our civic duty at the Fairmount Park in downtown Philly. She succeeded in communicating to us what a privilege it was to help out, improving the quality of life by picking up litter for six hours straight! So there I was with a smile on my face doing my good deed for the day!

During my high-school years, when children went to neighborhood schools, my high school decided to bus in Blacks from other neighborhoods, succumbing to the pressure to integrate. My parents believed that the unofficial segregation was unjust and fully supported school integration. "Everyone should be given the chance at quality education and quality medical care," they repeated over and over. As first-generation offspring of immigrant parents, they could easily identify with the struggling underdog of society. Without even realizing it, they had inherited the values and wisdom of the generations before, that pervading sense of justice passed down through the generations.

When I was in eleventh grade, my high school, Northeast High, adopted a "sister class" in a West Philadelphia high school whose students were Black and mostly poor. Once a week, we had a class exchange program and an end-of-the-year, three-day retreat. An excellent facilitator encouraged us to share our thoughts, feelings and information about our lives, in the hope that better tolerance and understanding would be created which would promote interracial harmony, and ultimately, world peace.

My mother was a staunch supporter of these programs, fully optimistic that social justice would prevail. My mom, bless her, was the ultimate hero standing up for justice. When we were old enough, we gave blood to the Red Cross where my mom volunteered giving out orange juice and cookies.

During my last year in high school, I knew exactly which field I wanted to work in: social work. I wanted to help people through struggles. I wanted to be a female version of Martin Luther King. Whether it was wayward teens, abused children, or the poor of the city, I would be there.

My father was diagnosed with colon cancer during my first year of college, with his untimely death nine months later. Attending a community college for a second year, I applied and was accepted to the Bachelor's degree program of social work at Temple University in Philadelphia. The university was not too far from home - my mom still needed me around- but far enough for me to feel independent. I had left home for a short period of time after my dad died to escape from the house. I had been thrown into the intensity of a mother-daughter conflict after my dad's drawn-out, painful death had taken its toll. I wanted out. Staying with waitresses with whom I worked at a restaurant, I would talk to my mom infrequently. I didn't know then but I would hold this guilt with me my whole life.

The practicum in the social-work field made my studies more interesting; visiting families in need, apprenticing with a counselor as interactive groups tried to solve problematic situations, was immensely emotionally fulfilling. I was thrown into the intensity of teenage issues of conflicts with parents and parents in turmoil about how to handle the rebellious youth. This was the heart and soul of what social work was all about. These were core, real, raw human emotions. It was problem-solving. It was helping people to help themselves. Book knowledge was important but working with people was my thing. I loved it all.

When I graduated college in 1976, I found a job working for the Philadelphia Department of Social Services, an agency that helped families function in a normal framework. We were to assist them in organizing their home and getting their kids off to school happily in the morning; to prepare healthy, nutritious food; provide clean clothing and show them how to balance their budget to cover their needs. These were poverty-stricken families. The task was challenging.

The first family the agency assigned me was the Rodens. I arrived and knocked on the broken door of an inner-city housing project, naively bright-eyed and optimistic.

"Come on in," said John. His black-toothed grin and his gravelly voice unnerved me, and yet I took my slow and tentative steps in.

I was immediately overwhelmed by the putrid stench that emanated from the living room. Despite the broken window which ostensibly gave 24-hour "ventilation", the odor was still wretched.

"Um… where is your wife Nancy?" I heard myself asking.

"Oh… she's at a neighbor. She'll be back soon," he said. "Why don't you have a seat, sweetie?" I looked at the food-stained, wooden chairs wondering which was worse, to insult him by not sitting down or to wipe the chair before sitting. Taking out a tissue to give a quick wipe, I sat down, thinking, *at least this skirt is machine washable*.

Two minutes later, Nancy walked through the squeaking kitchen door. At 4'10" and 160 pounds, Nancy's weight was hanging in a large, bloated, sagging stomach. Trying not to stare, I wondered if she had a serious medical problem.

"Hi there! You must be that lady from the agency," she greeted me in a friendly drawl.

"Yes, I'm Sarah. Maybe we can sit down for a while now to try to figure out where you would like to begin."

John pulled out from his back pants pocket a non-filtered cigarette and lit it. As soon as it was done, he pulled out another one. I coughed a few times, trying to breathe.

Pulling out my paperwork, I decided the first thing I should do before discussing a plan of action, was to ask for a tour of their home. They both readily agreed.

"Well, here's the living room. It's seen better days," Nancy said with a sweeping gesture towards the torn couch, the fabric unraveled and the rusted, broken springs exposed.

"This is what happens when you got two bouncy boys!" Nancy grinned in the direction of her two sons, a three and a four-year-old who were playing outside in the barren yard.

I heard the muffled, menacing growl of a canine barking, and asked, "Is there a dog around here?"

"Yes, sure is," John answered first. "We lock him up in the closet so he will get real mad. Then, if we go out or somethin', we let him loose in the house so he will bark and run around. Then no one will come in to steal anything."

I looked around the shambles of their home, honestly wondering what they had worth stealing, but I was trying to remain calm and non-judgmental. Inside, though, I was feeling anxious about being confronted by a wild, angry dog.

Then Nancy decided to take me upstairs. She showed me their sparse bedroom.

The old wooden beds were covered with torn, dark stained sheets. Again, I was hardly able to breath; the sewage smell that permeated the air was horrendous. She preferred not to show me the locked boys' bedroom. I agreed to forgo the experience, wary of what would be there. When we made it downstairs, the toilet-smelling house seemed more tolerable. I could begin breathing normally again.

The cries of a small baby became apparent to me as we entered the living room again. In the corner was a small once-white wicker crib. As I came closer, I saw the face of an eight-month-old baby with the body of a three-month-old. She was lying in a drenched diaper with flies whizzing around her.

"How old is she?" I asked. "Nine months old this week," answered Nancy.

"Is she okay?"

"Yes. She's a tiny one." Then while her husband walked to the next room, she whispered, "He sells food stamps for cigarettes. There's nothing I can do."

Three children's lives were at stake. I was

determined to help.

Returning weekly, with gloves to help while we cleaned and cooked, Nancy and I began to bond. It was an impossible struggle to help them balance a below-minimal budget. Their situation broke my heart.

The boys' bedroom had been a mystery for weeks and I was getting nervous and obsessed with the desire to go in. I wanted to attain the Roden's confidence and trust before requesting the key.

Nancy finally handed me the key saying, "Go ahead to the bedroom."

Walking in, my body froze as I slowly backed away. The bare beds and wood floors had defecation and the stench to match.

Clothes were probably in the small closet, which I was too fearful to open. Locking the door within seconds, I managed to make my way downstairs.

"Why does the boys' bedroom look like that?" I asked.

"Oh, well, we don't want them to disturb us in the mornings, so we keep their door locked until we are ready to get up."

I swallowed hard. With my eyes beginning to tear, I said I was leaving. I was tired and going home.

With mixed feelings, I reported the desperate situation to my boss. There had been little change in the cleanliness in the home, other than the days when I came. The food plan was not adhered to, the children ran wildly, unkempt and dressed in dirty clothing. They still fared poorly in school. Angry for the suffering of innocent children, I was enraged about the injustice. My boss had to turn the case over to the courts. They were out of our jurisdiction, beyond our ability to help. Immediate action needed to be taken to protect their children. This wasn't the first time there was a report on the Roden family. That's why we had entered their lives in the first place.

Two months later, I received a letter requesting my appearance in court, to report what I had objectively witnessed, to testify on behalf of the safety of the Roden children. The three children were placed in foster care. I prayed the family would get what they needed to be healthy and to heal.

In 1979, after only two years doing social work, I decided to pursue a master's degree. If I was going to learn for another two years, I decided it must be in a sunny, warm climate. My options appeared to be San Diego and New Mexico. San Diego appealed to me more, somehow. It was near the ocean and had one month a year of rainfall. Winter rarely hit freezing temperatures. And no snow. Snow was fun for skiing or sledding but not for shoveling the mound next to the car when I had to get to work. San Diego boasted winter temperatures of seventy-two degrees. My decision was made. Shangri La here I come!

My mom was fully in favor of her daughters earning a higher education. Though California was over 3,000 miles away, six hours by plane, visits were do-able. It seemed like such a drastic move, to continue my education so far from the East Coast. I recall one particularly sentimental night, once the decision was already made. I sat on the bed in the room that I had shared for years with my older sister. I mentally sorted through what needed to be stored and what I would pack to take with me.

Early September, in 1979, when I packed my bags, I sensed that I was on the beginning of a journey.

Greyhound had a three-day, cross-country $100 special. What a bargain! The rest of my savings I could use for food, rent and a trip back home sometime in the future.

Unable to eat breakfast, I packed some peanut butter on wholewheat bread for the long trip. I brought dried fruit and nuts, a couple of bottles of water and frozen orange juice. We packed ourselves - my mom and my sister Paula (Alice was at work) into the taxi, with my two suitcases and backpack. We arrived at the Greyhound bus station fifteen minutes before departure, which minimized the long goodbyes that I hated. With trepidation and some inner guilt, I kissed my mom's cheek. "Wish me luck!" I said after hugging each of them. I boarded the bus for my seventy-two- hour trip.

Could I really be leaving? I was just as stunned as they were. Wasn't I the daughter most attached to her mommy's apron strings? Wasn't I the one in the kitchen with her, helping prepare the holiday meals or looking for clothing sales, our favorite pastime? My mom's apron strings were loosening.

I looked through the bus window at my sister and mom standing on the platform. I smiled through the tears that welled up in my eyes, turning away as they began to flow. Nervous of the unknown, I focused on what I knew for sure: I had the youth hostel booked for the first week. After that, I had no clue where I would live, work, or who my new circle of friends would be.

When I reached my destination, I spent a week searching through the newspapers, looking for a place to stay. Before the first seven days of rent at the youth hostel were over, I noticed a small ad: a couple looking for a boarder for their three-bedroom, two-story home. I arrived the next day to meet my potential landlords. The home was in need of new side-boards and some internal repairs, but my room was clean with a nice multi-flowered bedspread. I was *crazy* about flowers. The salt-of-the-earth, middle aged couple seemed to be honest and hard-working. "No late night parties?" I joked after finding out about their structured days. "No, not us," they answered. It was close enough to the university, so I signed the lease, while we sipped mint tea together at the dining room table.

I soon found a market research job. It was more like soliciting, which I hated. I felt that I was bothering people trying to sell them something they probably didn't want, but it was a full-time job that paid the bills, and I needed to hang in there, until my studies began.

That spring, I took the required GRE (Graduate Record Exams) that I needed to pass in order to qualify to enter the university the upcoming fall semester. One month later, I was informed that the test results of the entire group of students were lost. As a result of this ridiculous development, there was no way we could begin the program that fall semester—we would have to wait an *entire year!!* I was engulfed with anger and disappointment. A quick appraisal of my life situation: I had no social life, a job I hated, and no money to visit my family and friends in Philadelphia.

Another full year? I couldn't. Holding the letter that bore the bad tidings, I collapsed onto my bed thinking, *There has got to be a reason for this crazy thing to happen! And I better see it soon. What am I going to do all next year? Where will I work? I can't stay at this job!*

Exhausted, but nevertheless trying to think of a solution to this situation, I fell into a deep sleep around 1:30 a.m. I didn't even call my family or friends to tell them the news that Princeton, the place where the exams were sent for grading, just added another year to my uncertain future.

When I awoke the next morning, I was able to muster up the courage to check the want ads, just to see what was there. More openings for secretaries (not interested), more phone soliciting (please, no), and a spot at a restaurant as a waitress. That was a possibility. I didn't want a sedentary job anyway.

Then, a couple of days later, about seven months after arriving in San Diego, I saw an ad which was exactly what I was looking for. The position was for a social worker at a Mexican-American youth center. I would be the assistant to the director. The drop-in center, which contained a pool table, ping-pong table and a couple of soda machines, provided counseling, job-search help and channeled the youth into programs designed to help them finish their high school diplomas.

I was hired two days after the interview. I relaxed on

the beach before starting work the following Monday morning.

The center was an over-sized ranch house on a hill top that attracted youth from various neighborhoods. This made for some friction. The gangs which formed among them sometimes had shouting matches. On weekends, when there was drinking, the end result was sometimes a swollen eye or puffy cheek, evident on the faces the kid's faces when they arrived Monday afternoon.

West Side Story came to life when I decided to bring the neighborhood gangs together on a project. Raising $1,000 from the local bank, I approached the less-than-proactive Mexican director about my idea of "the mural." He, himself, had been a graduate of the center so his main focus was schmoozing with the boys to keep them off the streets. He had no educational experience, so he left much of the directing to me.

I got busy contacting local papers for publicity for the center, rounding up a group of eight budding artists from four different neighborhoods. After three months, their center boasted a multi-colored mural of teens in Mexican cultural settings. The youth were so proud of themselves and especially of the group picture in the local paper.

In 1978, "Proposition 13" had been enacted. It was an initiative that added to the California constitution limiting property tax rates. This caused a shift in support for schools from local property taxes to state general funds. Unless I resided in California for at least a year, I would have to pay high tuition fees for attending the

State University which had been, until now, free for California residents.

After less than a year of working there, I had been promoted to official director. Now I had even less time for a social life. My life was the teen center. I wanted to start meeting people with whom I could develop friendships. I put my master's degree on the back burner. I had a job I was crazy about and wasn't interested in advancing my professional status.

A Mexican Jewish colleague at a liaison agency suggested I go to a local center for Jewish activities called Chabad. That was where he had met his fiancé. They are a world-wide group that helps Jews reconnect with their roots.

I immediately began to have a wonderful time meeting nice singles and warm families. After a few months, I decided to attend the local center's Torah (Bible) classes, and learn more about my heritage. There was hamantashen baking for Purim, those cute triangle cookies filled with jam or poppy seeds. They hosted authentic Passover seders for people to experience, supplied with huge round, handmade matzos, the likes of which I had never seen in my life. There were weekly Sabbath celebrations with beautiful festive meals, accompanied by the traditional wine and braided challahs. Not only was I intellectually stimulated, my heart was stirred. Over the following months, I slowly decided to stop working on Saturday, the Jewish Sabbath, a day when observant Jews do not work. Ultimately, this meant quitting my job on the teen center's busiest day. In the meantime, I took a temporary leave of absence. While attending the local Chabad house, I had heard about Manis Friedman's Women's Study Center in Minnesota and decided to sign up for the December session. It was a one-month intensive study program. Two months later I was airborne.

We were about thirty students, mostly college-educated women in their twenties from similar secular backgrounds. The classes covered meaningful topics, i.e., modesty in relationships, the beauty of the Sabbath, and laws between man and man. The information taught by dynamic teachers was both fascinating and inspiring. I was excited by being immersed for the first time in living a Torah lifestyle. I had been raised in a totally secular way, and now it suddenly dawned on me at age twenty-four I had a lot of catching up to do. Infused with a deeper appreciation of the relevance of Judaism to a modern life, I seriously considered moving to a larger, more cohesive Jewish community.

Upon returning to San Diego, I took what could be called "a leap of faith". With jittery nerves and a few prayers, I resigned from my position, sold my car and moved to Brooklyn, New York. I had been living every East-Coaster's dream in sunny California, with friends and family often saying, "How lucky you are!" or, "It's so beautiful there!" I knew I needed something more. People began to make comments. "Are you sure a cult didn't get you?"

My mother had been so proud of my decision to get my master's, and now I had to tell her these plans were on hold. I thought she would die from embarrassment. Here I was, returning to Brooklyn, the place my parents had escaped. *Plus-* I wanted to study Torah!

Just as I suspected, Mom didn't tell her friends for some time. She was very disappointed, yet we tried to maintain our relationship. There was an obvious strain because I had begun to keep kosher, so she couldn't cook for me anymore, and I wouldn't eat in just any restaurants. The Sabbath was now a holy day for me-- not a day to shop. And I was also very excited about my new-found religion. I wanted to talk about it a lot and I was hoping she would show some interest in the heritage that was both of ours. I wanted my family to understand me, but my enthusiasm was often expressed in the form of unintentional lectures, which turned them off. Mom couldn't believe that I wanted to learn and do any of this, as she had abandoned the little she knew about the Jewish way of life before she married my father.

To help make my visits more comfortable, I purchased some separate pots and pans to keep in a cupboard near her stove.

The movies and theater performances we used to share were now of little interest to me as I was trying to focus on learning about my new Jewish lifestyle. I preferred to use any spare time I had to read books on Judaism. That was of utmost importance to me now that I had adopted the traditional ways of my ancestors. Keeping the Sabbath meant so much but, now when I visited my mom, I would read alone after our Friday night dinner together while she closed the door of her bedroom to watch TV.

We continued to take walks on Saturday and play Scrabble, her favorite game. I tried to do whatever I could to find some common denominator to keep our relationship positive.

"I want to watch my TV shows on Saturday, not attend services," she declared.

"But Mom, it is such a special day for family; no weekday chores, and the best meals of the week," I pleaded.

"I know all about it. I had enough of this when I was growing up and I am not interested."

As a result of these painful new challenges to our relationship, my visits to Philadelphia were very few. We maintained weekly phone calls, where we tried to steer clear of sensitive topics and stick with general subjects.

Chain Snatching in Brooklyn

Excitement, passion and a sense of justice followed me to Brooklyn. In my mid-twenties, this was just another adventure to right a wrong and to save the world.

After making a decision to find my way back to my heritage, I found myself studying Torah in Crown Heights, New York, home to the Chabad Chassidim. After a brief stay of five months, before moving to Israel, I found myself involved in two robberies.

The first one happened when I went to a gym downtown. I got a cheap deal from a friend who had to give up her gym membership. The private lockers at the gym added another cost to my tight budget. Before leaving for the subway, I took some jewelry with me, and I left some at home, in an area I knew had robberies, even in the daytime. I had been renting a basement apartment with two other girls but no one was around in the day. Two of us were studying, the third working. The landlords, who lived upstairs, were mostly out during the day.

The rings, bracelet, and Krugerrand (a gold coin people bought at the time for an investment), I scattered around in different hiding places. I kept some in my jewelry box and a couple of other pieces in different socks. Returning after gym, I walked into a mess. The apartment had been turned upside down with clothes strewn on the floor, dresser drawers left opened and my new purple Fieldcrest washcloths blocking the toilet. It was an invasive robbery by not just ordinary thieves. My stomach churned as my eyes jumped around the tornadoed apartment.

My roommates' cameras were gone as well as jewelry from all of us, although some of my hidden items were saved. We called the police who came to file the report and assess the damage. "We can't do much lady, but here is a copy of the report if you need it for insurance purposes. If we ever find the cache, you may get your stuff back." Insurance? I thought. That's a joke.

As the days passed, I was filled with rage and humiliation. There were so many robberies and so many chain snatchings and the police were powerless to stop it. It was no wonder that when my friend, Michal, who was visiting me from nursing school in Miami, was robbed, I decided to take action. Wrongs had to be righted. That was my upbringing.

On our way to a lecture on a Sunday morning in

May, we were strolling down Eastern Parkway towards the community center. Chatting as we went, I suddenly heard a low, ascending scream from Michal as a guy came at her throat to snatch her gold necklace, which proudly bore her initial, "M". Taking off down Eastern Parkway, he ran towards Bedford-Stuyvesant, an area that a white girl just doesn't stroll through, even in the daytime. The relations between the Crown Heights' Jews and the Blacks in the surrounding areas had been very strained, but I wasn't exactly functioning rationally. My own personal feeling of violation was fresh in my mind. With my heart racing and adrenalin pumping, I ran after him shouting, "Call the police! I am going after him!". During the days before cell phones, my dad, may he rest in peace, always taught us to take a dime wherever we went. "You never know when you will need to make a phone call." Not having had a dime that morning, I left the apartment with a quarter.

Ducking behind cars and trees past row houses, which left me little place to run away if needed, I followed our robber until he arrived at a corner store, which boasted a sign, "We buy gold and silver." Diagonally across the street was a middle-aged Black woman talking on the only public telephone in sight. I was totally exposed in this neighborhood with nowhere to hide anymore. If the robber would come out of the store, he would see me immediately as the telephone hung from a pole with no booth around it.

"Please!" I pleaded. "I must make an emergency call. I will give you a quarter if I can use this phone."

"No problem. I'll hang up. Keep your quarter."

"Bless you," was all I could think to say.

911. The familiar number took five rings to answer. I was sweating from the run or the panic. They finally answered.

"I followed the chain snatcher!" (There had been a rash of these thefts for months causing girls and women to stop wearing necklaces or to walk in fear when they decided to wear a necklace for an occasion.)

"Please come. He is on this and this street corner."

Calmly, the lady on the other line asked, "What is your name?"

"Sarah, S-A-R-A-H!" Continuing with my maiden name and answering her where the chain snatching occurred, I said emphatically, "If he comes out of the store, he will see me."

"Hold the line," she answered.

Hold the line? Hold the line? Is she kidding?

"Did you just call from Eastern Parkway?" she asked.

"That was my friend whose necklace he stole. Can someone come already?"

The next two minutes seemed like hours when, suddenly, racing from three directions, were three squad cars with two policemen in each. Signaling to them towards the direction of the store, they motioned to me to come with them, I assumed to identify the thief. Oi vey. Crossing the street, we entered the store as I identified the only person selling gold that morning. He was handcuffed and taken away. After I gave a second policeman my details for the upcoming court case we would have to attend, I was almost ready to leave the store. I turned to the women sitting behind the glass windows, saying, "Is this how you have to make a living, from other people's stolen jewelry?" She stared at me like I was crazy.

The police drove me back to Michal who was anxiously awaiting my return.

"Are you alright? I was so worried."

Hugging each other tightly, I said, "Thanks for calling the police. You will get your necklace back at the court case."

Recounting to her what happened, she gasped, "The necklace wasn't worth your life." Still shaking, we walked towards the community center for a day of lectures on how we could serve G-d with our days on this earth.

I wanted to study longer but not in Brooklyn. I needed a change. Two robberies in five months were enough, especially after the court case when the police told me the robberies triple in the summer.

So, in 1981, I visited my mom for another farewell. I decided I was moving to Israel. My new lifestyle was hard enough for her, but the move to Israel threw her completely. I built up the idea of studying abroad gradually, but I actually broke the news one week before I left. Saying good-bye in person was important. I needed to show her I was sad about leaving as well as nervous.

I traveled to Philadelphia before continuing to Kennedy airport.

"Mom, I found this lovely place where some women go to study." I was too scared to tell her I was going but now was the moment of truth. "It's in Israel."

"What should I say?" Mom asked. The conversation, if you could call it that, was brief. That's all I remember.

I packed more of my "history" that I had left stored in Philadelphia, and boarded a plane for Israel one week later. My gut feeling was that I was not coming back. I told my older sister, Alice, but not my mom. This was 6,000 miles, not 3,000 miles away. That would have been too painful. Coupled with separating from family once again was the excitement of traveling to a country I had never even visited. A new chapter in my life was about to begin. I was twenty-six years old.

Chapter 3
Arriving in Israel

TAXIING UP THE summer green mountains of the northern area of Israel, I was enjoying my VIP service. People making aliyah (immigrating to Israel) were given a free plane ticket and a ride to their destination. Honestly, I officially made aliyah because I could not afford a ticket. The ride from Ben Gurion airport in Tel Aviv to Safed was a three-hour journey. Traveling during the late afternoon, I wanted to focus my half-closed eyes on everything possible. Despite jet-lag, I would enjoy my new adventure from the beginning. Some "highways" were the equivalent of streets in the small cities of America. Turning down one of these streets, traveling eastward, the driver veered away from the blue Mediterranean before the orange sun met the horizon. Twenty minutes up the road we suddenly stopped. My eyes scanned the area. What was the reason for this hiatus? I was a bit nervous about this detour. This man *was*, after all, a stranger, despite being assigned as my escort through the immigration department. A tent seemed to arise from nowhere. At the entrance appeared crates of red, light green and deep green apples. A short, middle-aged man approached with a cap on his head that didn't seem to have any effect in keeping the sun off his copper-toned face.

The stranger and my driver shook hands. It was obvious that they were friends. "Give me a case," the driver said. Pushing my suitcases aside as if the apples took priority, a case of large, red apples were plunked into the trunk. In broken English the taxi driver said, "Thanks for letting me stop. My wife loves these apples."

Shrugging my shoulders I said, "No problem" as he handed me one of the apples.

Arriving in Safed, 900 meters (2,953 feet) above sea level, was like walking out of a time machine. The cobblestone streets and centuries-old stone houses, almost completely destroyed after two earthquakes, were new or rebuilt in the original style.

The mountain air was so fresh, the town so quaint, I fell in love.

I explored the town with my friend, Lena, who had been learning in Safed for six months. We first met in Minnesota, but our paths were meant to cross again. It was comforting to arrive in a foreign country and find a familiar face. We frequented the bakery made famous because of their delicious miniature cakes and chocolate rolled pastries. The falafel restaurant drew a passerby with the smells of fried humus balls and French fries. The ice cream shop had three tables which seated two people each. A Baskin and Robbins it wasn't. There were about twelve flavors, not forty-eight. The shoemaker had a place the size of my mom's kitchen. It held the basic equipment he needed, nothing more.

Safed had a special atmosphere because historically this was where mystical teaching and liturgy were born. Before leaving the States, I had focused all of my attention on my learning.

My husband-to-be, Moshe, was sent to this town temporarily for work, and wound up being stuck there as his agency had no other placement for him to transfer to. There is a Yiddish expression, "Man plans and G-d laughs." I suppose he was laughing at my plans. My master's degree in social work was never to be. Moshe relinquished himself to working in his office and hanging out with the singles of the town, occasionally going out with a potential soul mate. While he was on a date, walking around the main street, our paths crossed.

One beautiful summer night with a cool breeze and stars so bright I felt as though I could almost reach up and touch them, my friend Lena and I were taking our ritual stroll around the circular main street. It was our "entertainment" of sorts as well as our exercise. Walking towards us, Lena noticed an old friend from her kibbutz days. Hanna's curly black hair hadn't changed. She was walking with a man, which among Orthodox Jews is either her brother or they were on a "shidduch."(date)

"Hello Hanna. How are you?"

As they spoke, Moshe and I just stood there, uncomfortably looking away. I was in seminary (a school for women only), a time when men and women did not intermingle socially.

Hanna called Lena on Sunday. "He is not the guy for me."

"Better luck next time. You are one closer," responded Lena.

About two weeks later during one of our walks, Lena and I spotted Moshe: 5'10", sandy- brown hair and green eyes, sitting on a bench on this circular street. He was, "coincidentally", there every night. Sometimes we would stop and chat with him. Our conversations were mostly exchanges about his urban planning projects in the North, and our Torah learning. After weeks of rendezvous' which lasted about an hour each time, Lena dropped out of our ritual walks. For her, it was enough to learn all day; she didn't need to talk about the classes through the evening, too. It was all new to me and I was ignited.

These meetings were not really permitted by my school. The "official" way to meet a guy was through a shadchan, a professional matchmaker. We only do that when we are ready to date. I was already 26 and a bit of a rebel so I by-passed this step. I wasn't even sure he was the guy for me. He was a distraction in a town with no nightlife and a listening ear while I shared what I was learning.

One evening, after two months of philosophical and personal discussions, Moshe, almost twenty-eight years old, looked down at his hands, folded one over the other. Noticing that he wanted to say something, I raised my voice asking, "What? What is it you want to say?"

"I want to ask you to marry me," he answered. Staring ahead into the dark night, all I could say was "Oh."

My mouth agape, and one of the few speechless times in my life, I said, "I didn't realize. Um, I have to think about it".

"Okay, then. Goodnight."

"Goodnight," I said, quivering, thinking, *what about*

my serious one year of learning? Okay, so I am twenty-six already. Maybe I should forget that and get on with my life: marriage, kids, a home. Was I ready? What have I done?

I called him two days later, asking to see him. We met near a bench, off of the main road. Taking a walk, I decided to ask him more serious questions. "You know, we need to talk about where we would live, what type of schools we would send our children to and other serious questions."

The truth was I was nervous because he seemed more serious than what I was looking for.

Suddenly, before we had a chance to discuss anything, a two-foot high pole was blocking our path in the sidewalk. He skipped over it like a little boy. It was adorable. It brought out a lighter side I hadn't seen before. That was it. Whatever else we discussed seemed less relevant at that moment. We parted ways after an hour, saying "See you tomorrow!"

Talking with my mom, Lena and my Rabbi's wife, Briney, about this major life decision and sharing my few hesitations, my mind was made up. One week later we were engaged. I flew to the States a couple of months later to show Mom pictures, tell her all about Moshe's family, and shop together for my wedding, something my mom dreamed of for years. At twenty-six, I was the first of my sisters to marry. Five months later, in February 1982, after Moshe's dad had recovered from an operation, we married in Safed.

Moshe and I settled in this quaint town where he was already working in his profession. As he worked, I attended classes, kept house and found some side professions to bring in some extra money. I bought a table top machine to make natural peanut butter. It was a big hit, mostly among the Americans. Israelis had an aversion to peanut butter because, during the 1948 and 1967 wars, it was difficult to obtain butter so the children were given peanut butter day after day.

My childbearing years blessed me with six children - three boys and three girls. My birth preparation course had given me confidence through knowledge, but it was Briney, my support person, who was my biggest asset. Briney supported me during my births. I originally met her by bringing her Skippy peanut butter from Brooklyn. Her mom was always sending care packages. There was one brand of peanut butter in Israel, but it wasn't Skippy.

Briney became my advisor and good friend. She taught me classes about Jewish marriage and had escorted me to the chuppah (wedding canopy). Briney, who had already given birth to three children of her own when I was birthing my first, helped me breathe and squat through my labor. We entered the hospital only when contractions intensified. The hospital was far from state-of-the-art, but I didn't know anything else. The two-bed reception room, called *receiving room* and *triage* in western countries, was the place where midwives assessed whether or not a woman was in labor. Broken water? Close contractions? At least 4 centimeters dilated? Once in active labor a woman went into the delivery rooms, if that's what you could call it.

There was a passageway leading down a huge room, with cubicles flanking the left side, each one having a door. They contained a birthing table, a monitor and a bit of standing room on either side of the table. The three-foot high walls, topped by a window, had simple curtains to give a feeling of separation from one birthing woman and the next.

There was no such word as doula then, only a concept of labor support. We ladies knew that women needed women to assist, especially in the Orthodox world of Judaism where there are restrictions on physical contact between husband and wife at certain times, including advanced labor. Moshe's role was saying Psalms, spiritually strengthening the experience. He would bring us cold water or refill the hot water bottle and in early labor he would emotionally and physically help me. I believed this experience belonged to women. It was about women supporting each other. Personally, I resented his look of sympathy when he didn't even understand what a period cramp was.

Briney was warm and supportive. Her encouraging smile and her strong hands were just the thing I needed to get me through labor pains at a time when epidurals were used for knee operations and hip transplants. It wasn't even in our consciousness to be drugged for birth. It just was not done.

I guess you could say that, except for in the Bible, Briney was one of Israel's first doulas.

Chapter 4
Turning 42 & Facing Empty Nest Syndrome

AT FORTY-TWO, MY youngest of six children was two and I was in a mid-life crisis. It's not that I didn't have enough to do with my life. There was my home to maintain; being a wife and mom is full-time work. We had also moved from our small mountain town, Safed, to Jerusalem. Although not New York, it was a much larger city than I was used to. For fifteen years, Safed had boasted 15,000 residents, a hall to host guest speakers, one movie theater, and seven "restaurants" (three of them falafel, two pizza places, one Italian, and by the time we left, a steak house).

The main hustle and bustle was in the summer when the tourist trade came to see the Artist Quarter and the old synagogues. Now I had to adjust to the big city with 620,000 residents, new traffic rules (seemed that anything goes) and familiarizing the family to a new neighborhood. There were new friends to meet and new schools. Adjustments took time. My family needed me. By the end of the first year, they had adjusted quite well.

Now, in our second year in Jerusalem my youngest was in nursery school and I was feeling an empty nest syndrome. There was no one at home from 8:15 a.m. until 1:30 p.m. Although all of my children still lived at home, I felt lonely.

There were very few opportunities for me to pursue a career. I didn't want a full-time job and my lack of good Hebrew-language skills limited my possibilities.

I knew that I still wanted to be part of a helping profession, but that's as far as it went. I was lost.

I tried to decide how to fill my days productively. I continued to bake homemade cakes and make soups from scratch, went back to Torah classes and joined a bi-weekly exercise class. To earn extra income, I juggled various jobs, including selling tofu and home-made natural peanut butter, despite the fact that Skippy had finally arrived in Israel. I also wrote my mom a weekly letter, occasionally enclosing the most recent pictures of the children. I created arts and crafts projects with the children, mailing them to my mom. She visited Israel every two years, and I had visited her as often as I could, bringing the newest baby with one of the older children. The children became our common denominator, which greatly improved our relationship. Now all we lacked was close proximity.

Toward the end of that first school year, sometime in May, an ad appeared in a Jerusalem paper that changed my life forever: **Labor Support course beginning in September. Help support women through their birth experience.**

Re-reading the main section of the ad, I thought *"Interesting. I had a good friend help me through my births. She was so supportive, so encouraging. She had a few children of her own. Guess she didn't need a title. I don't even know what a doula is."*

Anxiously awaiting Moshe's return home, I went for

a walk to release some energy. In those days, with no computer in the house, I couldn't even Google the word doula. How was I going to explain this to Moshe when I didn't even know exactly what this was about?

About 9:00 in the evening, when the house went into quiet mode, I sat down with an herbal tea, serving Moshe his new favorite brand of decaf coffee. The mood had to be just right with no interruptions. I switched the ringer off on the phone.

"So, what do you think?" I asked.

"About what?" he responded.

"Moshe," I said, pointing again to the ad. "Should I check it out?"

Reading the ad he says, "Sounds interesting. It'll only cost you two bus rides."

Wow that was easy! "Thanks sweetie," I smiled, giving him a hug for being so supportive of my ideas and various business ventures. I made an appointment to meet the teachers the following Tuesday.

The interview went smoothly. The two ladies wanted to know about my lifestyle. Did I have a support system? Did I have a back-up for when my husband wasn't around to get the kids out to school? What made me want to get into this line of work?

I began thinking about my pre-Israel life. "I know I want to be in a profession that helps people," I answered. "I also know I need a job with some excitement, action, adventure. There is no way I can have an office job. I hate sitting for any length of time. It's just not for me. Since I was sixteen, every job I had involved movement and action, whether I was a waitress or a social worker, with most time spent out of the office."

"My college years were spent in learning how to assist people through the Bachelors of Social Work degree I earned," I continued. They listened and I continued, telling them about my challenging but positive birth experiences. I shared how I had a "doula" friend named Briney, in whose bathtub I sat and food I noshed while in labor. "I want to learn how to do what she did and more."

"Thank you for coming," they said as they escorted me out of the room.

Chapter 5
Finding My Path & The Course

I WAS THRILLED when a week later I got the call that I was accepted into the course! We were starting in a month and I had a hard time controlling my anxiety. The month passed quickly. In anticipation of my new journey, I called my mom, my sisters and a couple of friends. The course was to be held in a local hospital. When Sunday came around, I walked through the hospital doors, finding the room where the class was held. After some paperwork and name tag preliminaries at the desk, we were ready to begin.

We were nineteen women sitting in a huge circle perched on bean bag chairs of all colors. We were a very eclectic group, ranging from age eighteen to fifty-eight. The former was an aspiring midwife, using this course as her springboard into the world of birthing, the latter a grandmother of eight who wanted to attend her daughter's births. Her daughter was in her second month with number four. Some of the students were religious while others not at all. Two wives of men working at the Dutch embassy were there to learn about childbirth while a divorced woman of fifty was there for a catharsis, wanting to heal after her two, and only, traumatic births over twenty years ago. She wanted to learn what could have been. And I was there to learn how to support women in the birth process. I wanted to give back what Briney, my friend who supported me, did for me. In a city which, at the time, was home to over 2,000 new babies a month. I was sure there was a need for doulas. Our one common denominator; an interest in birth!

As we opened our notebooks, we were introduced to a world familiar to some, strange to others. Carla, the inspiring midwife, had read many books on pregnancy and birth. The wives of the embassy men had not yet had children, and despite their being more than ten years Carla's senior, knew much less. We were all taking this journey together at our own pace. For me, I was searching for techniques and skills. I was also looking for answers to a global Truth. What is birth? Was it a medical event? Was it something spiritual? I knew that to "go forth and multiply" was a commandment. I learned that a long time ago. Why were women so fearful today? Maybe there was something about the way birth was being presented to the young women of this generation that made them go forward with trepidation. Even though I took prenatal classes and looked forward to my births, I hoped I would gain answers.

The anticipation of Sunday's class was more important than the long ride on two buses. In any case, I always carried a book about birth wherever I went. With pen and notebook in my tote bag, I would skip through the hospital doors, trotting downstairs where the class was held. This was normally the room where the childbirth education classes were held. One wall was lined with mirrors for the pre-natal and post-natal exercise classes; this multi-task room was sure being used wisely. This was where I would envelop myself in the womb, so to speak, for ten months. Little did I know how this time would revolutionize my attitude and spirit towards birth. Our group of women began forming friendships as the weeks turned into months. Some of us formed carpools while others connected to women who could back them up if they were too busy to attend a birth. I connected to Rina, a woman similar to me in many ways with an outgoing personality and religious affiliation. She would bring her emotional strength and faith in G-d to help the birthing mother.

The films on birth intrigued me. I stared at the screen, noticing nothing else. If I needed the bathroom, I waited, so as not to miss a moment. I had never seen a woman squatting or sitting on a birth stool while pushing. I had heard of the birthing-stool in the Bible but didn't think it really existed. I had no idea what it actually was.

In the 1980's, with the birth of my eldest, we were all reclining, many still on our backs. Episiotomy was standard while this lady on the screen didn't even tear! The baby's head crowned and slowly emerged. I stared at this film like others would watch an award-winning movie.

We learned the pros and cons of pain medication, episiotomy vs. tearing, what cesarean births entail, how to conduct prenatal and postpartum meetings and a wealth of birth information.

To me, this was it—life! Birth affects all people. I began to notice couples walking in the streets with their new babies. *Did they have a positive birth experience? Was she supported enough?* The emotional and physical outcomes have an impact that ripples like a stone thrown in a pond. We watched a film called *Labour of Love*. It was beyond the silver screen. It was real. It was the most exciting film I'd watched in a long time. Actually, it was probably the only film I had watched in a long time. And next to that birthing mom, was a woman, a doula, physically holding her from behind and encouraging her with soothing words, like "It's almost done. You're so close to seeing your baby. Soon you will be a mom."

So, as the course continued, I read and read. I read the eight required books and the fifteen optional. Janet Balaskas was the expert on water births, an option I never considered. *Immaculate Deception*, *Active Birth*, and *Spiritual Midwifery* were all new titles that I was introduced to. My kids began to stop asking, "Where's Mom?" They knew I was in my bedroom with a book on pregnancy or birth. I became the newly converted. There was nothing else to talk about or read about. I held myself back from calling friends and family because the conversation always led to birth. Frankly, not everyone was so interested. Some listened politely, while others just tuned out. Moshe got the brunt of it, so I tried to call Rina, my new-found colleague, who was experiencing some of these feelings, although not as strongly.

As the course passed the sixth month mark, we were encouraged to find clients whose births we could attend for free. On the bus, in the supermarket, and everywhere I went I saw pregnant bellies and I would ask, "Have you heard of a doula? I am taking a doula course and while learning, I am helping women as a free service. If you think I could enhance your experience I'd love to help." I left my number so she could think about it. I told friends, relatives, and neighbors. Slowly, women were taking an interest in the topic and in my services. In the meantime, our class had the opportunity to volunteer for eight different shifts in the hospital where the course was taught.

Birth without Borders

I encountered an unusual challenge as I entered the hospital to volunteer for an eight-hour shift one evening as a novice doula.

One evening into my fourth, eight-hour shift, I was hoping to meet a pregnant, fellow English speaker. It also would be ideal if she wanted a natural birth. Then I could practice my newly-learned skills! If she were an observant Jewish woman, I could support her through reminders of faith in G-d, and, on a spiritual level, help her get through the intensity of birthing her baby.

The one thing that none of our group wanted was to be bored for eight hours, waiting for a woman in labor to enter the delivery room. Sometimes, we had the disappointing experience of waiting for a woman to agree for us to assist her. Not every woman who came in wanted or needed help. Some ran in ready to push while others came in demanding an epidural. Once I saw a lady with a professional doula while others managed with their spouse.

I was told by the midwife that this shift was quiet, except for room #4.

Approaching the room, I took a deep breath in the hope that the couple would want some assistance and found a woman lying in bed with a long, black scarf completely covering her hair. She was wearing a long-sleeved plain blue blouse and had a beseeching look in her eyes. Her husband appeared to be twenty years older, as the grey in his sideburns crept through the black hair. Turning towards me, he asked, "What do you want?"

Standing in shock, afraid to offer my help, I said, "I am a student doula. We help women manage through labor." Taking a deep breath of air I added, "Would your wife want some help?"

"Whatever you can do, is fine. I can't stop her cries."

"What language does she speak?"

"Arabic."

"Is that it?", I asked him as we continued speaking in Hebrew.

"Yes. We don't teach them Hebrew or English in our villages. Some villages teach one or both. Our wives only learn Arabic".

I gulped. Okay, he could translate but *no* common language? And what if I say or do something wrong? What if she misinterprets what I am doing? How far do hand motions take a doula? She never took a course, never read a birth book. She was far from my ideal client for my first experience. It would certainly be an immense challenge.

"What is her name?" I asked.

"Fatma."

At least her name was pronounceable.

As Fatma's facial expression changed, I realized a contraction was beginning. I exaggerated my breathing, bringing my face close to hers, so she could follow my lead. When the contraction waned, I gently held my arms out to her hands, motioning for her to bring her legs downward to the floor. I thought she would be better standing through the next contraction. One thing is very clear from my learning: birth was meant to be active and upright with women standing and squatting.

Fatma followed my lead, swaying her hips as I did. I handed her husband a washcloth requesting him to wet it to cool her brow.

I could barely pronounce his name. "Call me Jake," he said after a while.

So, Jake and I were bringing nineteen year-old Fatma into an unknown world of birthing her baby. She was compliant and followed my lead as I gave instructions with my eyes, hands and heart. I prayed I was going to help this mom birth her baby, sans trauma.

While I continued massaging and applying back pressure, she changed from upright to rocking on fours, helping alleviate her pain. Gently holding her by the shoulders while staring into her eyes, kept her focused as she was handling each contraction one-by-one. Her eyes would meet mine as we breathed through each contraction together.

Wiping her sweaty brow, a sign that she was advancing in labor, I was relieved. Then suddenly, the next few contractions brought a look of panic in her eyes.

Watching her reach her hand behind her back, towards her bottom, I asked Jake to ask her if she wanted to push. Calling the midwife, her pace quickened to our room, as she heard a major scream. Asking Fatma to come onto the bed, the midwife was pleasantly surprised to see a head crowning. She gave instructions when to push and when to rest. These words midwives learn in most languages.

A robust, 3.5 kilo baby boy was born. Fatma cried. Jake sat down in shock. As Fatma's mother walked in the room minutes after the birth, I left the family to revel in their experience. A short time later, Jake walked out to return to work, thanking me profusely. Helping a birthing mother without even a common language made me elated and invigorated. If I could help this mother, I could help anyone! I left the hospital thinking that I had truly found my calling. The year 1998 was proving to be an exciting year.

Chapter 6
Mom's Diagnosis of Alzheimer's

AS I WAS on my journey into my new profession, my mother started her journey, albeit a downhill one. One day, my older sister Alice was visiting mom. After playing a game of Scrabble, my mom's favorite, they took a walk when my mom suddenly said, "Look at those nice raw flowers." My mom realized she had said something wrong. Alice knew too but decided to chalk it up to old age. It was clear she meant wildflowers not raw flowers. Old people do that a lot. Nothing to worry about. Alice tried to rationalize, but inside, Alice was concerned. Denial can be a calming way to deal with the inevitable when there are still no other symptoms.

Alice had signed up for the Peace Corps that summer, so she left. After returning to live with my mom during the Christmas break from the Peace Corps, there were more signs. Checkbook balancing became an issue. A pot of boiling water was forgotten on the stove until they smelled smoke.

Alice decided to have mom tested. The doctor didn't come back to them with the results so, assuming there was nothing to report, Alice returned to finish the year in the Peace Corps with a nagging feeling inside. My younger sister, Paula, lived a mile away so Alice felt Paula could keep an eye on Mom while she was finishing the year in the Peace Corps. A few months later, when Alice returned, my mom was re-tested to confirm what the doctor suspected- Alzheimer's.

Over the next couple of years, Mom made only one more trip to visit us in Israel. She and my sisters needed my support. It came through phone calls and letters but once every two years I would continue to fly there, usually bringing one of the kids.

Five years into Alzheimer's, Mom's speech became more confused. She began to speak less because she had more difficulty finding the words. She was angry at her friends who called less and rarely visited. When I spoke to them, they admitted that being around her became more frustrating. Conversations became more difficult and going out for lunch became more embarrassing when she forgot words or behaved in a childish way in public. The library for the blind stopped calling her to read books onto tapes. The Red Cross, where she volunteered for thirty years, called her less frequently and eventually stopped completely.

Craving to be the most professional doula I could be and the best daughter too, despite my personal and professional commitments back in Israel, I decided to try to visit more often. As Mom's Alzheimer's progressed and even though my *seemingly* independent, teenaged children really needed me more emotionally, I would visit yearly. I was increasingly torn between my obligation to my family and to my mom.

Once I arrived in the States, I attended conferences related to birth, juggling that with the guilt of leaving my mom, even though they weren't far from Philadelphia. I was also leaving behind clients in Israel who might give birth before I returned. At least these conferences helped me to recertify while giving me a distraction back in Philly.

"What date will you be back?" asked a long-standing client.

"June 8th," I answered. "I know. It is two weeks before your estimated due date."

"I always go early," she answered, with anxiety in her voice.

"I know, but never two weeks," I said. "And just think, I'll already be up at night with jet lag, so I'll be in an ideal position to help you!"

I gave my clients a feeling that they were the most important people in my world. I would drop nearly everything in my life when they were in labor. And I did! I would cancel doctor and dentist appointments. I put appointments with new clients on the back burner because a woman in labor was first priority. Short of my own child's wedding, I could be counted on. If two births collided, I had a back up, an absolute must.

In the early stages of her disease, my mom herself had said, "Keep the plane money for your family" or "Your husband and kids need you more than I do." I went anyway. I knew she really wanted me to come. On one of the trips, I went with her to a memory group at a center for older people. The facilitator gave tips on how to retain words and how to sharpen the brain. Crossword puzzles were good but my mom's favorite was Scrabble. I played with her every day and she usually won. She knew all those two-letter words that I had never heard of.

When we returned home from the center during this last visit, we practiced making lists and memory associations. It was interesting and helpful, but I silently cursed that my mom needed to go through this. She could still play Scrabble, but by my third visit, five years into the disease, it was getting more difficult. The words she tried so hard to create were in her mind, stuck there. That was when I had decided I had to come yearly.

Chapter 7
Meeting a Client

A PRENATAL ENCOUNTER is a time when a client interviews me to ascertain if I could be the right doula for her. Women usually hear my name through a friend who has used my services; word of mouth is really the best recommendation possible, much more effective than advertising, business cards and even my website.

Our first encounter is usually brief—about thirty minutes to discuss what the woman needs to have a safe and positive birth experience. She asks what is included in my fee: phone calls, pre-natal visits and even a false alarm when we have gone to the hospital only to be sent home a couple of hours later.

Discussing the couple's birth plan, I inform them of how I can help them meet their expectations.

Meir and Lisa were sent to me by a previous client. During our first meeting they were very sure of what they wanted. This meeting took over an hour.

"We have read a lot of books and spoken to friends," they said.

Lisa was the most vocal. "I am in the middle of a childbirth preparation course. Meir works too many hours at his new job, so I review with him on the weekends."

I let her continue. "We don't want interventions done to us and we want a part in all decisions."

"Okay, fair enough. Unless it is a life-and-death, immediate decision, you should be involved."

"We want you to tell the nurse not to break my waters, for example."

"I will remind you of what you wrote in your birth plan. I can be your advocate but not your voice. I will help you make decisions regarding any interventions, telling you the pros and cons, but the two of you will have to make the decisions with your caregiver."

These prenatals are also a time for me to sense if I think the "chemistry" is right for me, too.

At a second meeting, we discuss the methods they learned in their childbirth education course. We practice some positions, go over the breathing method they learned and I show them techniques and comfort measures with which I can help them.

Turning to Meir, I ask, "How would you like to participate? When would you like to be involved?"

"I don't know. I've never done this before," he answers.

"I am not there to take your place but to work as a team. You can assist her for a few hours, calling me when you begin running out of ideas or losing steam. In the hospital there are ways you can help too: bringing drinks, refilling the hot water bottle, and praying."

This is a time for connecting, a time for them to share any fears or concerns they may have.

This is when I have an opportunity to say to Lisa, "If there is anything you'd prefer sharing with me privately, woman-to-woman, you can call me this evening."

I have had calls from a woman saying, for example, "I am afraid of internal examinations. I have heard they are very painful." I assure her that I can quietly share this information with the midwife, so that she will avoid doing any unnecessary examinations and certainly try to be gentler.

A large dose of intuition is essential as a doula—during these meetings as well as during the births. I remember having met a couple whose husband was very quiet, for example, showing little or no enthusiasm during the prenatal. Taking note of his demeanor, I asked if he had questions that we were not addressing. He then expressed his hesitation asking, "Why is it necessary to have a doula? Haven't women been giving birth for centuries without any help? Why do we need to pay for this now?"

"Very legitimate question," I say, validating his feelings. I then provide the vital statistics of the documented benefits of having a doula, which usually appeases the partner's concern.

During the prenatal encounter I also inquire if there are any medical situations that I would need to know about that may affect her labor or delivery. For example, symphysis pubis is a condition of joint separation that the woman would usually benefit by pushing lying in a side position.

There are other concerns that may require attention or referral to professional consultation: for example sciatica, migraines, joint swelling, hair loss, excessive nausea. She may need to consult with an herbalist, a physiotherapist, and/or other complementary healers for long labors, pelvic-floor issues and more.

Information such as this is usually not provided by a busy staff in a socialized medical system and even in a country like the United States, when women enter a shared practice with a few doctors.

I also encourage prenatal exercises and reading material appropriate to the couple. For example, if she is having a VBAC (Vaginal Birth after Cesarean), I highly recommend a couple of excellent, informative VBAC books.

These prenatal visits are a wonderful opportunity to build up a woman's confidence while establishing a connection with the couple during this highly charged, transformative time.

Chapter 8
Challenges in a Medical System

AFTER ATTENDING SOME doula and midwifery conferences in the States, many times I returned frustrated that I wasn't experiencing the "ideal" birth. Although there were some improvements- men were now allowed in the delivery rooms and our cesarean rate was still much lower than the States- there was so much more that needed working on. It was a real challenge going back to work while remembering the midwives from the midwifery conference and the doctors and educators at the doula conferences. Reading all the research also made it frustrating to return to work in a medicalized system. It brought back memories of my own births in hospitals, when the traditional shave and episiotomy was done without question. It was a given, like most new moms in the 1950's who dried up their breast milk because they were told it was best to bottle feed. Research had proven that routine episiotomies were *not* beneficial. They were even *detrimental*, introducing bacteria and infection.

These professional highs and lows coupled with the frustration of Mom's issues were unnerving. Deciding where Mom would eventually live and who would be the primary power of attorney of her medical, financial and physical affairs was still uncertain. We would have to watch and wait.

Still, I believed hospitals could offer a positive and safe birth experience. Most women wanted a skilled doctor who supported their desires as well as someone skilled in obstetrics. In Israel, midwives attend each birth so the experience is very different than in other Western countries. A skilled hospital midwife, attending the delivery, is routine. If one is fortunate to get an open-minded hospital midwife rather than someone who was stuck with out-of-date beliefs, the birth could be a positive experience.

On one of my visits to the States, I met an ob/gyn who told me, "The hospital staff has the pressure hanging over them of a potential malpractice suit. This affects the decisions we make on how to handle a birth." I read this in a book I discovered by Jennifer Block called *Pushed*. Very objectively written, she explains, "Obstetricians have behind-the-scenes pressures which have nothing to do directly to the delivering mom. As the doctor told me, 'Personal pressure also weighs in with some of our professional decisions. Rising malpractice insurance is forcing obstetricians to even leave our profession.'"

In Israel, women have the option to hire a private doctor in the hospital while private midwives can only be hired at a homebirth. There were three home-like birth centers in Israel and in 2003, hospitals began to open in-hospital birthing centers. The majority of the hospital-employed midwives were trained with the medical model of care, i.e., continual fetal monitoring, and routine amniotomy (breaking the water bag). However, they have now started attending advanced midwifery classes which offer traditional midwifery approaches including a natural and holistic approach to birth. They include evaluating the emotional state and history of the birthing mom.

Childbirth courses, now attended by over half of expectant moms, give women confidence to speak up for themselves, and more recently, the benefits of doulas have caused an increase in a doula-accompanied birth.

Sometimes there was friction between how the midwives were handling the progression of the labor and how the general doctors on the floor wanted to handle the birth. A doctor would walk in to analyze the situation by looking at the monitor strip and the midwife would say, "She is already nine centimeters!" Well, keep me posted," turning on his heels.

Some of the men or women in green work well with the midwives and others want to take charge, making final decisions. On the totem pole, the doctors do, in fact, make the final decision. We, the doulas, are definitely low man on that totem pole, probably even one step below the cleaning lady. The friction between the midwives, many who have had twenty years of experience, and some doctors, some fresh out of med school, can bring tension into the delivery room. With one trying to respect the other, there are some dialogues and exchanges which can leave the doula in an uncomfortable position. So, when this happens, I attempt to shrink into a corner or focus on the birthing mom as she copes with the labor pains, pretending to ignore the staff dynamics. Recently I experienced a "shrinking violet" day as a birth brought the caregivers to a wrestling match of who would topple the other. I will call the doctor Cobi.

Let me describe the delivery rooms. They are standard. Like many western models, some of the equipment is hidden behind cupboards or curtains. The entrance to the room has a door which is always left open for quick access. About two meters in front of the door is a ceiling to-floor curtain, allowing for modesty as the traffic ebbs and flows in the room. As the curtain only nearly reaches the floor, we "visitors" are privy to who enters the room if we recognize their shoes.

As my client progressed to complete dilation, with some occasional decelerations on the monitor, the doctor wanted to know if she was ten centimeters yet.

"She is 9 ½," answered Devorah, the midwife. "I will be able to raise the cervical lip soon." Devorah suggested I lay her on her left side so the decelerations are less frequent. Glancing at the clock, the midwife was biding time as she knew the doctor was one of those control freaks with less experience than her. He would be in the room any minute to deliver the baby by vacuum if she got to full dilation and remained there longer than he deemed medically acceptable. Unfortunately, doctors are usually called in to see the emergencies. As it was clear in *The Business of Being Born*, a must-see documentary on birth in America, most doctors have never seen a natural, vaginal delivery. In this particular hospital, cesareans and vacuums are the highest in Jerusalem. If it weren't for these midwives, it would be higher.

Now, about fifteen minutes later with full dilation,

we saw the doctor's shoes at the space between the floor and the curtain's bottom. The midwife instructed the woman, "Push as hard as you can because I see the baby's hair!" (I was internally cheering the midwife on as my palms began to sweat). The midwife glanced over her shoulder, towards the base of the curtain, to see if the doctor was walking into the room or would hear that she was pushing and walk away. She gave me a wink and I whispered, "Thanks so much." The contest can be unnerving. I was grateful that the birthing mom wasn't noticing the dynamics.

An eerie feeling came over me, looking at the feet under the curtain, as my mind brought me to another one of my life's adventures about the town thief. His feet too, were seen underneath my long living room curtain as I awaited his entry.

When we lived in Safed, that mountain town in the northern part of Israel, there had been a thief, robbing houses of unsuspecting moms as they picked up their children from preschool or kindergarten. Most of us left our doors unlocked, as there hadn't been a robbery since we could remember.

During the colder months, I hung a curtain in the inner section of our two-foot corridor entrance to block the breeze when someone entered the house. The bottom of the curtain didn't reach the floor.

One day, resting on the couch after a morning of housecleaning, there I saw them. A man's pair of shoes peeking out from under the curtain. The robber!

"Think fast, I said to myself." Not knowing if he was even armed, I called out, "Hello. My husband isn't home yet. He said he would be a bit late."

"Okay," he answered.

As he left, I grabbed the phone. "The thief is in my house. The Safed thief is in my house!" Giving the police directions, I hung up the phone, going outside to follow the thief. I looked everywhere for signs of the police as I ducked behind cars so he wouldn't see me following. Turning his head, he saw me.

As he dashed, I ran. Across the road I saw a police van coming and waved my arms frantically, pointing to the thief as he darted down a hill. The police shouted "Get in!" So Starsky and Hutch pursued. Others were on the hunt so someone caught him further down the road. They whisked me to headquarters to identify my intruder. Our town had been saved.

My mind returned to my birthing mom.

She pushes out her son with a high Apgar score. There is a cord wrapped around his neck. "Cords are wrapped in as many as 30% of births," says the midwife. "If needed, we bulb-suction the baby and lift off the cord, placing baby and mom together."

Mom and baby lay together, baby wrapped securely in her mother's arms. Mom stared lovingly as she raised her eyes to the father of this child saying, "We are parents. Here is our baby." They lay claim to this moment and this birth. In their own space, all is quiet, peaceful, and healthy.

Rescuing a town from thieves is one thing- women shouldn't need to be rescued from birth.

A Faucet of Blood

Excitedly dialing a colleague, Julie, I am happy to hear her "hello."

"Guess what?" Giving her no time to answer, I continued, "I am reading an insightful book called *From Doctor to Healer* by Robbie Davis-Floyd and Gloria St. John."

"I think I heard of it," she replied.

"It talks about the basic models of American health care- the technocratic, humanistic and holistic paradigms. She follows the thoughts and feelings of *forty* physicians as they expand their horizons in order to offer more effective patient care."

"Okay," she said and continued to listen patiently.

"They learn a mind/body separation model with the patient as an object and technology/science as paramount. I can understand how a doctor can have trouble relating to me when I ask that a client be allowed to stand/shower/eat and drink through labor."

"Great insights," said Julie.

"Honestly, I used to feel anger or occasional pity but now I realize that I need to speak their language and have loads more patience. When the client has been put in a passive role I also have to speak to *her* about taking responsibility for her pregnancy and their baby. Is there a reason that the nurse has to help her weigh herself or put the dipstick in her urine cup? This is a two-sided affair."

"You are so right! Can I borrow it when you are finished?"

"Of course," I answered. "Have a great day!" Click on the other end.

Then I began to ponder.

When, for instance, at a birth center a pregnant mom is involved with her nutritional care, charting her weight gain and using the dip stick for her urine evaluation, she automatically assumes more responsibility for her baby's and her well-bring. A team effort has proven to be more successful in providing for a healthier pregnant mom as the evidence indicates by fewer premature births, normal weight gain, and higher Apgar scores.

For me, part of my learned patience in this profession came from Shellie Moore. In January of 2002, Shellie Moore, a DONA doula trainer, came to Israel to facilitate a DONA (Doulas of North America) workshop. She impressed me as one of the calmest doulas I had ever met. She exuded that all-important trait of patience with her smiling blue eyes and soft-spoken voice patiently answered our questions.

Shellie was from Washington state; pristine and quiet. Our two-day course was short because the group had some knowledge. No detailed explanations were needed to explain terminology or physiology for birth. We sailed along. Pictures were taken, addresses and farewells shared. Within a year of meeting all the requirements, I became a certified DONA doula, my second certification. My sister, Alice, sent me a dark purple lab coat. It had wonderful deep pockets for carrying some needed supplies for easy access. Purple is the color for relaxation. Lavender is the aromatherapy oil of choice for many women. It is always a color that I favored. It helps my clients and even the staff stay "chilled out" when a situation becomes tense.

A couple of years after this second certification as a doula, I met Dr. G., Michelle's private doctor.

Michelle called me from home with a scared voice stating, "I am bleeding. Not just a little either."

Knowing Michelle was only thirty-six weeks, we are dealing with a premature baby. "Go to the hospital immediately. Call Dr. G. on the way to fill her in. I will meet you there."

Shutting off the partially cooked stew which was to be our family's dinner, I called a cab. Grabbing my birth bag and a bottle of mineral water, I paced outside waiting for my ride to come. In five minutes it arrived. I told him, "Don't get a speeding ticket but I am really in a hurry." We pulled up to the main entrance of the hospital in fifteen minutes, rather than the usual twenty-minute ride. Bless that driver.

Running into the delivery room, I caught my breath and watched the scene unfold. My first encounter with Dr. G. was in delivery room number eight, when we converged on our mutual client as she experienced an abruption of the placenta, a life-threatening situation for a fetus whose oxygen supply is detaching from the uterine wall. Delivery had to be immediate or the baby would die.

Placental abruption is also the main cause of maternal hemorrhage. I had never witnessed a placental abruption. I took a deep breath, saying to myself *Get hold of yourself. You need to help Michelle now.* I tried to draw on my learning to calm the atmosphere amidst the emergency.

I took Michelle's hand. "Breathe with me. It will give more oxygen to the baby". She was already breathing through an oxygen mask. I smile as I tell her, "You are in skilled hands. Dr. G. is doing everything that has to be done." Michelle's husband asks, "What is going on? Will everything be alright?"

"G-d willing," I answer. "They have to work quickly."

Another doctor ran into the room asking if he could help. "Call the pediatrician," ordered Dr. G, taking charge of the situation.

Almost mesmerized, I saw this petite doctor, latex gloves in hand, shouting, "Bring in forceps; she is fully dilated." Blood poured out, and there was no time to monitor the baby. Dr. G. delivered a thirty-six-week-old baby girl. She handed the baby over to the midwife who placed her on a warmer bed to be observed by a pediatrician.

Dr. G., wearing jeans and a tank top as she accomplished her rescue mission said, "I was out walking my dog when the beeper went off. I only had time to wash my hands. Sorry about my outfit."

I was so touched with her consideration of this religiously-observant couple. Dumbfounded, the couple and I, although dressed in long-sleeved blouses and skirts below the knee, didn't know whether to laugh out loud or not. We were so concerned about the mom and her child; none of us had even noticed her clothes. I decided this was a special lady, someone I was hoping to work with in the future.

Four months later I met Dr. G. again in a different setting. I wasn't sure how she would work with a low-risk woman. In the prenatal meetings, she agreed to monitor the baby intermittently. I was told by others that the women who hired her have freedom of movement, take showers, and eat and drink as they desire. Everyone knows their place in the birthing room, including the doula who is there to support the birthing mom. However, the doula had leeway when working with Dr. G. There was mutual respect between the doctor and doula. Dr. G. had the final say when it came to medical decisions; however, if the doula questioned a procedure, Dr. G. listened and explained. The doula was also given the liberty to make suggestions if the baby was not descending or the labor stalled. Dr. G. was receptive to position changes, nipple stimulation and other techniques a doula might suggest.

When standing next to some of the male doctors, Dr. G. exuded a confidence that assured me she is their equal. This may have taken time to develop, but to the doulas, despite her short physical stature, she stood taller than most of her peers.

Our mutual client, Miriam, a primip (mother birthing for the first time) had been in labor fifteen hours by the time we entered the delivery room. She'd been in labor nine hours at home before she called me at 1:30 a.m. asking that I come to her. A few hours later, we were off to the hospital. The fresh morning staff welcomed us as they had just replaced the night shift who left at 7:15 a.m. red-eyed. "Eight births last night," they told me, "and others are still in labor. They more than earned their day sleep." Dr. G. arrived an hour after being called and was told that Miriam was seven centimeters dilated. Refusing the offer of pain medication, Miriam asked Dr. G., "Can I return to the shower?"

"Sure. The monitor looks fine. Enjoy."

I helped Miriam set up a big blue birth ball in the shower. "Can I have some quiet time to myself?" Miriam asked. I brought the CD of relaxation music into the bathroom and closed the door. "I am right outside if you need me," I called as Miriam's husband left to the synagogue to pray the morning service.

When Dr. G. returned to the room she greeted me with a much appreciated good-will gesture. "Here, you look like you could use this," as she handed me an Earl Grey tea bag. I suppose I looked more tired than I felt. "Thanks so much," I responded as I filled a cup with boiling water. Another hour passed. "It is really time for a quick monitor," Dr. G. requested. "Maybe we can see how she is progressing." I knocked on the bathroom door. Miriam agreed to come out only if she could return to the shower. "No problem," said Dr. G., "Let's just see how the baby is doing."

Ten minutes of monitoring showed the baby was alright. Dr. G. let her stand, making the contractions more manageable. Miriam headed back into the shower saying, "I don't want to be checked now."

"Okay, just don't push in the shower," answered Dr. G with a grin.

Sometime later, Dr. G. returned, wanting to check her progress.

"She really wants to stay in the shower. Is it possible you could check her in there?" I asked.

"Only if you turn off the shower. I need these greens for the next few hours."

"Will do," I said, filling in Miriam.

"Almost ten centimeters. It's time to come out. Delivering in the shower is not my style. Sorry," said Dr. G.

Drying off, Miriam put on a fresh hospital gown. I was busy wiping her forehead with a washcloth and giving her ice cubes to suck. "I want cold, anywhere and everywhere," she pleaded.

I used my plant mister to spray her hair and back. Her husband filled it up every now and again with more cold water as it emptied.

Allowing Miriam to push on her knees facing the back of the bed, Dr. G. said, "Can you turn around now so I can have better support of the perineum? The head is crowning."

Red-cheeked and sweating despite all the cold, Miriam cried, "Whatever you want. Just let me keep pushing!"

I supported the back of her neck as I helped her hold up her legs. Miriam and I took one more breath pushing together as she brought her baby boy into the world.

"Not a tear," said Dr. G.

With doctors like Dr. G. there is hope for having the skill needed to assist in an emergency and a hands-off approach allowing a woman to birth her baby as she needs. I also see a light at the end of the tunnel that maybe doulas will, one day, become part of the maternity care team.

Chapter 9
Singing in the Rain & Moving Mom

MY MOM'S SIXTH year into Alzheimer's, she reached a plateau and then she began to decline again. She began to use the word "thing" instead of the correct word. Many times she couldn't think of the idea she wanted to convey so she said "It isn't fair."

"Don't worry, Mom. I'll wait until you think of it." Little comfort, I am sure.

I tried to help her complete her sentences or searched for the idea she was trying to express. I decided to try to look at the bright side of our time together. I would make the ten days we had as fun as possible. I would try to find humor even in the trials and tribulations even as I watched her deteriorate.

On this plane ride I closed my eyes remembering last spring when I flew to the States.

One day on a shopping expedition, rain was predicted. Assuming we would return before it began, we went to the shopping center a mile away sans umbrellas.

Returning on the regular city bus, a twenty-minute route from the mall to Mom's house, ominous clouds appeared in front of us. Passing red-brick twin houses as we headed through Northeast Philadelphia, the ride was taking us straight towards the storm. No umbrellas. No raincoats. Light sweaters and a few purchases in paper bags with handles.

"What do you think, Ma?" I asked.

"Doesn't look too promising," she answered with her eyes looking forward through the driver's huge windshield window.

"Well, there's no turning back."

Knowing my mom has strong legs from walking miles every day I said, "We will have a brisk walk when we get off the bus."

As we inched closer to the corner of her street, the two-block distance to her house suddenly seemed much longer than usual. We disembarked from the bus as the drizzle became a downpour, suddenly becoming torrents.

"Come on Ma! We can make it!"

We tucked our handbags under our sweaters, and continued our trot. I grabbed my mom around her elbow and forearm, crossed the street, stepping into an overflowing gutter. About three minutes to go! We jogged up the long cement driveway, cracking from years of neglect, and I started to sing, "I'm singing in the rain, just singing in the rain, what a glorious feeling. I'm happy again." Dancing around my mom, we began to laugh, knowing there was no way to escape. "Mom, we are soaking wet and running won't help." Laughing, we slowed down our pace. A large puddle loomed before us in the driveway. I jumped right in the middle of it like a little kid, joyously sending splashes in every direction. "We are dripping anyway, so what's the difference?" Looking at me with a grin as if I was a silly child, Mom removed her key from her wet pocketbook, opening the basement door that led into the laundry room.

Throwing our outer clothes into the Maytag, we draped ourselves in towels and headed for our rooms to put on dry clothes. Putting the kettle on, we sank into the couch cradling two steaming cups of tea, still laughing at how silly we must have looked acting like children in the streets. I doubt that anyone saw us but if they did, I didn't care.

That had been a special trip. This one, however, was much harder. This trip I found Mom was not in such a good mood. It worsened when the subject of her leaving her home of thirty years came up. I was saddened knowing that she knew she had to leave her home. She was against the idea of going to an old-age home because she did not feel old. In her mid-seventies, Mom was given no alternative. Although she always said, "I won't leave Bergen Street except feet first," it was not a possibility now. We were concerned for her safety. None of her caregivers were dependable or had been to Mom's liking. She also refused to pay, "Just for someone to sit and watch TV with me?" But after burning a couple of kettles, forgetting what she went to the store to buy, and losing her ability to count change, Alice and I decided Mom could no longer live alone. She was a danger to herself. Paula, my younger sister, wasn't in total agreement. She was uncomfortable with the decision because she knew our mother's heart was not in it.

After a slow-moving Scrabble game, which I purposely let my mom win, I decided to bring up the subject of moving. I had to convince my mother (and myself) that it was a good idea because she could still live independently and have fun. "Mom, you won't need a live-in. No one will be in your space. You'll have activities and people to talk to, a van to take you shopping. There will be movie and game nights."

In mid-winter of 2002, Paula and I took my mom to

investigate three old-age homes. Alice was working full time. This wasn't easy for any of us. We decided on the one closest to her neighborhood. The lobby was warm and welcoming with early American furniture and sofas that she could sink into. It was Mom's style and the area was familiar to her.

"You will be a short bus ride from your favorite shopping center!" I said. Mom was actually starting to look forward to it or maybe, given no choice, she was convincing herself that it would be alright. And it was— for three months.

Then the complaints began. The phone calls kept coming and I was sleeping less. I was agitated that I lived so far away. Mom was angrier each call. "The women are catty." "Film night is nice, but I've already seen the films at least twice in my life." "Entertainment night is silly." "The walk-for-exercise is not for me." My energetic mom, who so enjoyed walking, still had a pace much quicker than the group. Needing no walker or cane to guide her, she trotted way ahead of the rest.

I remembered her shopping trips to buy all the non-groceries. The little enclave of fifteen stores flanked by Gimbels and Wanamaker's was about a mile away. Granted, most of the terrain was flat. She trotted the one-mile distance in less than half an hour. Passing our one-story, sprawling, elementary school, veering past Dunkin' Donuts, she sometimes waited for the light to turn green as she made her way down Bustleton Avenue. Well, at least the home was only a bus ride away.

But now, she was fed up with the "old biddies" in Paul's Run. Mom always felt younger than her peers. So, with trepidation, three months after the move, I flew to the States to visit her.

Moshe understood the seriousness of what was happening with Mom, but it was still hard to run the family alone. He was my best confidant. He would overhear my phone conversations with my mom. Speaking slower and clearer than ever before, I said, "Mom, Tsippy is graduating college. College. She is finish-ing four years of un-i-ver-si-ty."

This is how the conversations went. When I hung up, I cried and Moshe gazed at me lovingly, handing me the tissues. Those were the times Moshe was around and within earshot. Otherwise, I stayed locked in my bedroom alone. Taking a deep breath, I returned to the kids as if nothing had happened. I had to be brave, had to be strong. Letting me fly became easier, at least, when I returned with clothes and toys. I could not yet share the seriousness of my mom's condition with them. I didn't think they were ready. Maybe I was the one who wasn't ready.

My sisters' disagreements over how to handle mom's situation frustrated me. It became worse when I saw it first on my visits to the States. They rarely agreed on anything, from doctor's appointments to caregivers. This trip, I registered for a "Midwifery Today" conference. I thought this would raise my spirits.

Ina May Gaskin, the famous midwife from "The Farm" in Tennessee was going to be there. It is exciting being surrounded by midwives, my modern-day heroes. I feel so beneath them as they are so knowledgeable, strong, caring. They are the salt-of-the earth who believe in the process of birth. When I am with them, I feel I want to be in their presence forever.

One thick-accented woman, recently relocated from Africa to America, explained how to birth a breech baby vaginally. Simply put, "the bottom comes down, reach in to bring the legs down. You don't have to worry about asphyxiation because you place your fingers in the baby's mouth flex the chin to clear the nasal passage and the baby can begin to breathe already."

When I asked how many episiotomies she had done, she said, "One and that was on a vertex (head down) presentation."

"How many damaged babies?" I asked.

"One out of over two thousand and I am not so sure he didn't have in-utero problems already. We didn't have monitors or ultrasounds." As I watched her, my mind flashed back to high school. She reminded me of a teen I had met when we were trying to promote interracial understanding. She was strong, determined and smart.

This midwife continued to demonstrate how the widest circumference of the head above the ear can be slowly brought down to stretch the perineum just as with a vertex baby. With my mouth agape I watched her demonstrate. "No need to cut," she said. "It's as simple as that." She'd done it hundreds of times because half the women from her town in Africa birthed breech babies.

One day, after the conference ended, I returned to my mother's apartment to find her sitting in her coat, gloves and hat. After a minute of trying to find out why she was dressed to go out and why the apartment was so cold, she looked up at me blankly. "Why haven't you turned on the heater?" I asked as I walked over to the unit on the wall. I realized she didn't understand how to turn on the heat. "I am so cold," she complained. "What is wrong with this apartment?" She asked as if the managers were to blame for the temperature.

When back in Israel, I received a call from Alice telling me that Mom (who was still able to navigate the bus system), got off at the wrong stop and wandered around for several minutes looking for her new home. She finally stopped in a church to ask a priest for help in locating Paul's Run. He called and let the staff know that my mother would be "home" shortly and took her back.

When the staff director sent a letter, voicing his (and the staff's) concerns that my mother could no longer live independently and would have to be moved to the assisted living facility part of the building or leave, I knew we'd reached rock bottom. According to him, she wasn't eating, did not know to dial "911" in an emergency, and could not locate the emergency button. When my mother was confronted with these challenges, the excuses started: "It's different from what I'm used to." "I never knew how to work the emergency button." She had many more excuses to justify the tragic reality: her mind was going.

My sister called again. "The home, in no uncertain terms, wants Mom out of independent living. She is a danger to herself. In the assisted living unit, Mom will be locked behind doors. Even if they are made of glass, Mom doesn't want it."

"What are we supposed to do?" I asked.

"Well, she didn't say it emphatically that she would

not go there," Alice continued. "She just stared at the glass doors that one has to be buzzed through, as if they were iron bars of a prison." The "tour" exposed the people inside for what they were; stripped of their freedom, downsized to rooms which fit a bed, dresser and closet, the last stop before nursing care or the "next world."

"I remember when we first toured Paul's Run," I told Alice. "When we came to this section, Mom's jowls seemed to lengthen; her eyes lost any semblance of feistiness. My heart sank watching her, watch the "inmates."

A caregiver was the only solution. So, still in the home, with four months on the contract to go, we decided to finish out the year. While I had been in Philadelphia, I hired a part-time caregiver, Mary. Mom hated her. We soon discovered that she was doing what *she* wanted to do, including watching TV programs that *she* wanted to watch. Now the agency tried to send my mom others but frankly, the double payment of a home and a full-time caregiver seemed like a waste. The two other women we sent were not to my mom's liking either. We also had to make sure her funds would last. So, we decided an apartment with a full-time caregiver downtown near my sister, Alice, would be the best solution.

The worst thing for an Alzheimer's patient is to keep relocating. My guilt set in once again. "Sorry, Mom, but look at it this way; you always liked movies, theatre and restaurants. Everything will be just down the block from you *and* you'll be closer to Alice."

She thought it was a great idea. She was fed up with the home and the people who resided there but she was mostly fed up with herself. Sometimes she held her head saying, "I want a new brain." I don't want the phone with the large numbers to press." "I don't want someone to live with me, just give me a new brain!" I flew in three days before the move to help her pack and adjust emotionally. While there, she screamed about her brain again.

"Mom, I am so sorry. I wish I could give you one."

I wish modern medicine could take away those horrible plaques but they can't yet. I hugged her tightly. Inside, I shuddered knowing this could be genetic.

Three months after her move downtown, the complaints began. The excitement was wearing off. Her part-time caregiver, Karen, who Alice had hired before the move, was very responsible and caring. She agreed to become a six-day live-in. Karen was off on Sundays which made part of Alice's Sunday's permanently booked from lunch time through dinner. Alice made sure Mom had her meds, food and even worked hard to explain "Sixty Minutes" Sunday evenings. Paula rarely came. She was busy with her teaching, which required loads of after-school lesson-planning, test grading, and phone calls to parents as well as parent-teacher meetings.

I think the situation was too emotionally hard for her to handle. Reality set in when we realized Mom could no longer go to the theater. Movies were out too. They are "too loud," the people "talk too fast," and "I don't understand what is going on." The rare times Alice took her, she spent the whole time explaining to her what was happening, while people keep shushing her or giving them dirty looks.

Conflicting calls came from my sisters like "Mom's fridge is half empty. She has no food." The other said, "How much does a seventy-year-old woman need?"

My stomach was in knots. "Moshe, I can't stand this anymore. Mom needs better supervision. Paula was too busy, even on weekends. Alice was fed up. We had to think of another solution."

Those flights, the past two years, had left me on an emotional roller coaster. I hadn't figured it out yet but something strange had been happening when I returned home, trying to get over jet-lag and catch up with life. It's true that there were e-mails and phone calls to answer so there was the stress of that. I also had to struggle with putting my power-walks on hold, while in the States, because Mom needed me and she certainly couldn't walk as fast as she used to. Our walks had been reduced to around-the-block strolls.

Returning to Israel after a visit with Mom, I started walking again but a black cloud was still over my head. My children were doing well, my husband had a job and we were all healthy, thank G-d. So what was it? Why did I feel like crawling into bed and not coming out for hours at a time? I was in a depressed state about what I left in America but it dawned on me that I needed the "high" of a birth! Yes, that was it. I was obsessed and addicted.

I hadn't had the adrenaline which permeates the room when a woman is in labor. How did I know? Because when I got that first call after being off the birth scene for a couple of weeks, my whole body shook when hearing her voice. The rush, the high, the blood, the sweat, the fluids, the baby's cries. I loved it all. Some people are addicted to drugs, others to food, cigarettes and to alcohol. I was addicted to birth. Two weeks was much too long to be without one.

Marlene's eager voice was on the other end of the line. "Hi. I think I am in labor. I have been having pain in my back since this morning and it is coming every seven minutes."

"How are you managing? What are you doing to cope?" The conversation continued for fifteen minutes while I timed her contractions.

"I will call you after a shower, as usual, when it gets a bit closer," she added.

I double-checked my birth bag. My mood began to swing upward. Hot water bottle-check. Aromatherapy oils-check. Massage tools-check. Relaxation music- check. Granola bars and cold water bottle- check.

I waited outside for a taxi rather than order one. Usually, when I called one taxi to come to the house, five taxis passed while I waited anxiously to get to my client's house. I gave Moshe a quick call to tell him that I was on my way to a home birth with a mom I had been with before. It was even more exciting because homebirths were a rarity. As of the writing of this book in 2014, with about seventeen homebirth midwives in the Homebirth Midwives Association, they comprise less than 1% of births in Israel. The government does not subsidize them yet, so many women, who would consider a home birth, cannot afford it. Actually, for all the prenatal care, postpartum visits as well as being on call for the birth, their price is more than fair. Most of it goes to insurance and taxes anyway.

I arrived to see Marlene dancing around the room to rock music. I left my music in my bag. She was gyrating in a way I hadn't seen since the late 60's. I thought, *Whatever works for her. We are going to have a blast.* The midwife arrived an hour later to join the fun. Laughing as Marlene danced, we sang to the tune as if we were a band. The poor midwife, trying to monitor the baby's heartbeat, jumped to Marlene's pace asking her to hold still after the next contraction. I tried to press on her back while I ran around the room in sync with her. In and out of the bath for a twenty-minute spell, she kept moving in the tub too. Three hours after I arrived at Marlene's house, she caught her son while lying in her bed. A birth! That's definitely what I needed to pick up my mood. And this one was just what the doctor, or in this case, the midwife, ordered.

Chapter 10
Why Women become Doulas

WOMEN BECOME DOULAS for various reasons. I decided to interview two colleagues, now friends.

A Celebration of Love
"Chava, why did you decide to become a doula?" I asked.

"Originally, a friend suggested that we become doulas because we both didn't have children yet. Living in Jerusalem where we were surrounded by women who were raising large families, we were constantly reminded of our distressing, painful circumstances. Her great idea was motivated by the fact that both of us had been married for several years and Naomi thought this would be our "in" to the mysterious, illusive world of pregnancy and birth."

"Really? Didn't you think it would be too hard working with pregnant women, when you yourselves becoming doulas, we'll have something to offer, we'll know didn't have any?"

"Yes. I thought it was a crazy idea, and at first I was very resistant to her grand plan. I told Naomi numerous times that I wasn't interested, that this would be too painful. She totally disagreed and convincingly retorted, "No, Chava, this will be our in! By what everyone is talking about. We will have our own "birth stories" to be part of the inner circle, instead of being stuck looking forlornly from the outside."

"Naomi so succeeded in winning me over to this worthy cause that I ended up offering my centrally-located home for the initial meetings."

"So how did you feel once things started to get underway? I asked.

"Well, one noticeable change in our home was that we now had plenty of inspiring birthing books in our apartment. I also became alerted to the potential risks of unnecessary and sometimes dangerous medical routine hospital interventions. This heightened my awareness of the need to help protect women. I really did start to feel "in" on the subject, that I would actually have something to offer, even if I had not (yet) given birth."

"Were there other influences in your life that made you open to going in this direction?"

"Yes, definitely, I can credit my mom. My appreciation for the natural process of birth was enhanced by own mother's exceptionally positive attitude. She gave birth in the sixties, in the era of "twilight" medicated births, where women weren't even aware of what was happening to them. She was a pioneer!"

"Then what happened?"

"Well, this is going to sound unbelievable, but the first birth I attended was when I was twenty-seven years old, with a neighbor who heard that I was interested in becoming a labor coach. Sara was willing to depend on me for support even though the course hadn't even started! She was already past her due date when we spoke, and her birth ended up being induced."

"How did it go?" I asked

"Even though it was a difficult, medically managed birth, I was totally in awe of the entire process that she had welcomed me to witness, and I cried freely when her big baby boy was born. Incredibly, within two months of this landmark event in my life, after over three years of marriage, we were expecting our first child! We canceled our next appointment with the adoption agency where we had been attending regular meetings about this option."

"That is amazing! Then when did your actual training begin?"

"It was the first offered in Israel, way back when hardly anyone had heard of the concept. It was organized by Leah Marinelli, who is now a midwife in Monsey, New York. Back in the late 1980's, when Leah made aliyah with her family, she was surprised that there was hardly any awareness of the benefits of labor support. She took all her enthusiasm and belief in a woman's ability to have a positive birth experience and did something about it! She searched for a midwife, and discovered Aliza Levine, a knowledgeable homebirth nurse-midwife, who was willing to teach us. Leah organized the students; she came up with a name, and IMA—the Israel Maternity Association—was born. (Now, her practice in Monsey is also titled IMA for Informed Maternity Alternatives.) There were about ten students, the course lasted over six months, our required reading was very comprehensive, and we all loved it!"

"So you were pregnant while you were studying to be a doula?"

"Yes, there I was, overwhelmed with gratitude that I was actually expecting a baby, when I began this intensive training. The information Aliza taught with her warm vivacity and positivity filled me with a wonderful sense of anticipation for my much longed-for birth. We chose to have a homebirth with Aliza. I was fully aware of her admirable competence, and trusted her reliability."

"So, this sounds like it was a life-transforming, turning point in your life."

"Yes. My passion for helping women have positive births is greatly influenced by my personal history, especially assisting women who struggled for years to have children, or underwent other birth- or life-related trauma. A positive birth can be extremely healing."

"Anything else you would like to add?"

"Well, don't let me forget to mention that my friend Naomi also eventually had children, thank G-d!"

Becoming Me, Becoming a Doula

"Anna. How did it all begin, your enthusiasm and your passion?"

"It started 16 years ago, but I still remember the feeling in my eyes - swollen and heavy. Somehow I managed to open them. My vision was blurred but slowly the image of my husband sitting at my hospital bedside became clearer and clearer. His face was etched with worry, but a small smile grew on his lips as he saw me trying to focus on him."

'Anna…' he had said- half question, half statement,

'You're over it, you gave birth!'

"I knew I was supposed to be happy and excited. After all, we were talking about the birth of my firstborn, but I was too nauseous and exhausted to even smile. "What did we have?" I whispered. I was so depleted of energy I could barely talk."

"'A girl, she's beautiful, I saw her!' he replied trying to garner some enthusiasm from me."

"I rolled my head to the side; the tears had started to flow again. I felt neither happiness nor accomplishment; rather, I felt disillusioned, let down and sadness so great that my body shook as I sobbed. My whole body felt bruised and abused, I couldn't move without waves of pain crashing through my mid-section."

"I had just been through 24 hours of induced labor in the hospital, constantly berated by midwives that my baby was too big to be born from below. I was chastised for being "so late" (I was two weeks past my due date). I was bullied into pain relief I didn't want, forced to take an epidural that actually was put in wrong and didn't work, and secretly given a medication (Pethedine) I had asked not to be given. I was kept lying down for most of my labor, and it's no wonder that after 24 hours my birth ended up in the operation room where they prepared to slice out my baby. I would have understood if the operating staff had listened to the midwife who told them that my epidural had not worked and I was without pain relief, but they did not bother. They cut anyway. Finally they administered a general anesthesia so I would be completely out – and quiet."

"I am so sorry. Go on," was all I could say.

"Later, as time went by, my feelings were replaced with an anger that grew and grew inside of me from the depths of my belly which had been carved open in order for me to birth my firstborn. The anger bubbled and rose inside of me for months after my birth, swirling around my head and heart. As time ticked by, the cloud of anger started to settle but what was left was strength so great I hardly recognized myself. As my new baby daughter learned to smile, roll over, crawl and walk, I too found myself becoming a new woman. I was strong. I was capable. I was prepared. I was never going to give birth like that again!"

"The initial steps of the journey that led me to becoming a doula were for personal gain and becoming a doula was not even something I had thought about. Simply put, I knew I wanted more children, but I would never again take birth lying down! I had a plan. I reeducated myself on how the body works during labor. I learned that negative input ("your baby is too big, too late"), stress and the supine position all hinder the birth process. I would come to my next birth armed with confidence, education, knowledge and a *doula* – my personal positive support person! Had I known about ICAN (International Cesarean Awareness Network), I would have had even more strength."

"So you heard about a doula this time around?" I asked.

"Actually, it was mentioned in the childbirth preparation course my husband and I took, but we seemed prepared enough to go it alone," she mused.

"But for the next birth, you changed your mind?"

"Yes and eighteen months after my first birth the night finally came for me to call her. I whispered the words I had been looking forward to saying for the last few weeks, "I am in labor." I had already been awake for several hours with contractions, but this time I embraced them rather than feared them. I welcomed every one as a step closer to my baby. I imagined my body as a rose bud, opening up to reveal my new baby inside. I watched the stars traverse the sky wondering when my baby would be birthed into this world, calmly and gently as I had always wanted, and just like my body had been created to do."

"When my doula came at around 5:00 a.m., she immediately reassured me that I was strong and capable and that this time I would have a better birth, even though some circumstances were the same. I was again carrying a big baby. I was again two weeks past my due date. As the contractions grew more powerful and as they washed over my body, my doula helped me stay afloat. I was strong, I could do anything!"

"It must have been an amazing feeling for you," I said, validating her feelings.

"After watching the sun rise over the mountains, which was my view from my house, we arrived at the hospital. I greeted my midwife and after some brief paperwork, I let her check me. Amazingly I was already minutes away from my baby, I was almost fully dilated. After three pushes, I birthed the plumpest baby I had ever seen. She was bigger than my first. She was bigger than the baby they had to cut out because they said she was too big to be born from below. All along until this birth I instinctively knew I had been wronged, I knew there had been nothing wrong with me or my body – and now I had the proof! I had previously had an unnecessary cesarean. That day I could have danced for hours, I knew such joy from giving birth - as women had been created to do - that nothing could keep me from beaming and laughing all day! My body worked!"

"Within a few weeks ladies started to call me to ask how I had managed to have such a good, uncomplicated birth. Ladies stopped me in the street to talk. I was like some kind of secret heroine. I had managed a quick uncomplicated VBAC, with no need for pain relief to boot! I gained knowledge from support groups on the internet; I networked and then started to go to birthing conferences in my city. I helped one, two, then five women have better experiences in the labor room with my telephone advice before labor, and my fame was growing!"

"My ability to have uncomplicated and easy labors became the talk of the town with each child that I gave birth to. By my fourth child my husband would joke that I was the neighborhood birth consultant. My mind was made up: I would become a doula to help other women become empowered, to trust their body, and come to enjoy birth as I did. I would encourage them to become pro-active in their decisions in birth and labor. I would help them gain self-confidence and I would show them why birth can be an uplifting emotional and spiritual experience. No woman would have to face the trauma and disgrace of the medical world as I did that one night several years earlier. No woman would come away without feeling something positive about her birth process. Even babies who needed to be born from above could give their mommy reason to be happy. There would be no such thing as a traumatic birth if I could help out!"

"Nine years after my cold, sterile and painful birth, I embarked on a doula training course which propelled me into the labor room. Before I had even completed the course, I accompanied a woman on her first birth. She had a typical first labor, long and slow, but with no need for pain relief. I remember how beautiful she looked, the colors in her face as she breathed and swayed through every contraction. I made sure to tell her how well she was breathing, how she was glowing and how she could birth this baby. She was strong and confident, just as I had encouraged her to be. She birthed a healthy daughter. We all cried together, they for the joy of a healthy daughter, me for the satisfied and whole mother that had been born, along with her daughter. Walking away from this birth, I had a smile on my lips and my heart sang. My journey had just begun."

"Thanks for sharing," I responded with tears in my eyes. "Keep up your great work!"

Chapter 11
Choice, What Does It Really Mean?

I OFTEN PONDERED the word "choice." Words can be very subjective as they are influenced by our environment. From the suffragettes to the modern-day woman, choice is what is spoken about. We doulas have to support our women (couples) in their *choice* in the labor process. In some years, books about women choosing to reduce labor pain (with drugs) or having elective cesareans because of convenience (many times from fear of birth), evoked sadness or anger in me. There are so many women who are ignorant of their own potential.

Labors are begun or augmented (sped up), in 50% of births in America and approximately 30% in Israel. How are women expected to choose non-medicated births? (I have attended inductions which were non-medicated because my ladies were motivated and the inducing drugs were raised more slowly than protocol.) Vaginal births after cesarean (VBAC) are occurring in just over 10% of subsequent birth after a cesarean in America while in Israel, women achieve a VBAC in over 80%. Sadly, even the method to deliver breech babies is not in the medical school curriculum anymore, anywhere.

Where is the true free choice in these births?

After reading books and seeing films which have

exposed the "business" of birth, I understood the options that women have and don't have. When we give women the supposed options of different drugs for management of labor pains, on what are they basing *their* choices? On what are they basing their views of birth? I have read that much is based on the dramatic TV shows which depict birth as something frightening. It's also from stories they have heard from women who have been traumatized from their managed births. My good friend, Michal, became a midwife. She worked in L.A. for a couple of years and she described births like this. "Vaginal suppository is given at night to induce labor. By morning the doctor adds Pitocin, breaks the amniotic sac and delivers quickly through instrumental delivery and episiotomy. Hopefully the mom will be at forty weeks."

"How did you handle that?" I asked. "It was my job. Those were the doctor's orders. If I didn't like it, I had to leave but, at the time, I had nowhere else to go."

Is that how we understand birth? And how about viewing this from the birthing mom's side of the situation? Does society give them tools to prepare properly for one of the most momentous times of their lives?

What happened to eating the best foods, exercising for a healthier baby, reading books that inspire as well as inform? In addition, is the system supporting women for a healthier and safer birth? Are there truly choices offered to cope with the pain? There *are* some practitioners and hospitals in America and Europe who have updated their methods of practice, and in Israel we are going towards an awareness of natural births with fewer interventions, more homebirths and additional in-hospital birthing centers being built.

Are we near to DONA's mission statement: "A doula for every woman who wants one"? This support system makes birth much more manageable and reduces request for pain medication. While we are creeping closer, we are still far from it. Even in hospitals which have showers, I hear over and over again that women are showering to cleanse themselves, not for pain relief. Most women are offered an epidural as the only mode of pain relief and readily accept it. Most women are still lying down while strapped to the monitor instead of standing, which is more painful and slows progression of labor. Most women are still not supported during the birth process, something that many "primitive" cultures offer, but Western ones are lacking. Ironic. "Nothing by mouth" (No eating or drinking during labor) is still an old idiom being used in the year 2014.

In a time when every negative experience needs to have a quick and easy fix, why are we allowing this to be carried over into birth? Who said birth was meant to be easy? As Kathy McGrath once said, "Birth is meant to be overwhelming. It is a life-changing experience." (Thank you, Kathy.)

As I tell my clients, we are meant to be challenged beyond where we think we can go. We are meant to tap into our emotional and physical strengths. We are meant to ask G-d for the courage to go on. It is a time when we go from "having a mother to becoming a mother" (Thanks again Kathy) and being a hero is worthwhile. Carrying and birthing a baby is a privilege and an honor.

Birthing with courage and strength can help us to handle *life's* pain and challenges.

In Genesis it says, "In toil you will birth." Things worthwhile in life are more appreciated when they are achieved through hard work. Is this work ethic gone forever?

Let's rise to the challenge. Let's climb the mountain and feel the adrenaline rush as we reach that peak!

It is true that some of us are not meant to climb that mountain. For personal reasons, having a baby is enough for them. And that's okay. But, if we have a friend who is feeling down, would we think it is important for them to choose an anti-depressant as a first option? Wouldn't it be better to vent with a friend or a professional, take an exercise class (which stimulates positive feelings), take a vacation or other numerous alternatives? Should we, as doulas, support someone who wants to choose medication as her first choice? The analgesia enters the bloodstream and crosses to the baby, albeit in small amounts. And we speak about **choices**: how about the baby?

The baby is not making a choice regarding his willingness to be medicated. The increase of fetal distress, failure to progress, use of stimulating drugs and forceps/vacuums for the delivery is well documented. Are we there only to support the mother, even if it is at the expense of the baby, even if it is *her* baby?

I am in a dilemma. Should we support a woman's choice to opt for pain medication before the first contraction comes? After interviewing women, they often tell me that this "choice" is based on negative birth stories friends have told them. The fear is not coming from deep within her through knowledge or experience. I always advise women to keep an open mind and try, for the sake of herself and her baby, to have the healthiest birth experience possible. I have seen the other side, too. I have witnessed how an epidural has helped a woman greatly in the progression of labor. There is a place for medication, but it is more rewarding and healthy, in my opinion, if a woman first tries without it.

A few years after becoming a certified doula, for the second time I attended a first-time mom's birth who was told, "birth is too difficult and for you, it is not doable without pain medication; i.e., an epidural." The woman added, "Even my mother told me to take one as soon as I can." She attended a childbirth education course that encouraged, inspired, as well as informed. The mother-to-be really wanted to try without pain medication. Contractions began at 8:00 a.m. We had phone contact most of the day until at about 3:00 p.m. it really started to get difficult. I arrived to find her coping fairly well, but she was definitely at a point that her husband was running out of ideas and stamina. "Lets' try different positions," I said. I also helped her to do visualization. "Would you like some music for relaxation?" I filled the bath. We stayed at home until I saw that she was beginning to truly fall apart. She didn't want to arrive early because, once in the hospital, the temptation for an epidural would be too great. Arriving at nine centimeters, she delivered her baby in less than two hours.

When she phoned her mother, her beaming eyes and

the excitement in her voice exuded confidence and thrill. "Mom, I did it without an epidural!"

The power of support, information, and physical assistance really can make a difference.

I feel the need for doulas to be supported, share information and receive positive strokes.

More networking should be done among birth professionals.

TALI: Doula Support and Professional Advancement

Summer camp. A sorority group at college. A tour across Europe with a small, guided group. What do all these things have in common? The thrill of being there, the high, and the let-down when it is over. When an intense emotional group experiences something so positive, there is the elation that deep in one's core pleads, "Do not let this end!" The bonding wants to continue forever, cemented with super glue.

That's how I felt at the end of my first doula training, in 1998. There were nineteen of us in that group and the energy surged. We became involved as we practiced massage techniques on each other and brainstormed as to how to handle a stalled labor. We began to know each other from something as basic as what food we brought when it was our turn to share the brunch, to the deep exploration of our emotions regarding our own birth experience, including a loss of a child. We laughed, cried, and had a lot of fun together. This course catapulted me towards my future career. It became a passion in my life and I wanted to share my learning and my heart with most, if not all, in this group. Not everyone continued on my path, and of those who did, not everyone felt this electricity surging through their bodies as I did. There were other women out there attending births and I wanted to know them all. I wanted to meet periodically, sharing birth stories, information on upcoming conferences, new books or research out there in cyberspace. I felt the need to fill the emptiness of the end of my training by creating a forum for doulas to learn together on a regular basis.

After some investigation, I was surprised to discover that there was not yet any forum that existed in Israel. Early in 2003, I phoned some classmates who were equally as enthusiastic. The responses were varied when I asked them if they would be interested in participating in ongoing meetings. Some lived too far away to participate regularly, but told me that I should e-mail them about upcoming events. Some had large families, while others had part-time jobs.

I asked the teacher for the list of women who were not in my class. I phoned another doula trainer for her list as well, even though she taught only every few years. Unfortunately, the latter never kept her list of students.

Then I began gathering up women's names from contacts I had as well as the names of childbirth educators and lactation consultants. Slowly, I amassed a list of over seventy doulas.

The next task was to update their contact information. Somehow, I was never the "One Minute Manager", a great book that I should have re-read before taking on this project. The project went something like this: Ursula's number, out-of-order; Karen moved out of the country; Rebecca, the same; Nancy, no longer worked in the field. This is how it went until I whittled the list down to fifty doulas. That was enough as far as I was concerned. My family was getting fed up with the phone calls. I had to leave messages when there was no one at home, so I received as many calls as I made. I tried to dial as the front door closed with someone leaving and hang up when I heard another family member walking down the front path.

Now, where to begin? I thought. I had better invite a guest speaker to bring in the busy ladies. Most would take time out of their schedules if the magnet was strong enough. I began with a homebirth midwife. My thought process went like this: women who believed in homebirth would come because they knew Ilana or believed in homebirth. Others would come because they knew nothing and wanted to learn. Yet others would come to network and see what this was all about. TALI, (Hebrew acronym for Doulas of Jerusalem) was born, so to speak. I never knew how many doulas would attend and if we would meet the speaker's fee. Forming this group was a risk worth taking!

I learned quickly that I had to take into account women who could not come because of a child not well at home, an appointment on the day of the meeting, and, of course, a birth. I decided to take the chance.

Splashing on some Shalimar perfume, my mom's favorite and now mine, I was off to the first meeting. Pouring into the huge living room of a woman from the group, were women who I knew and others I had never met. Some names were familiar from a birth chat group on the web, so now I could put faces to the names. This was going to be fun! Thirty-three women came, mostly doulas. The room continued buzzing for twenty minutes until I could speak. Women were meeting each other for the first time and others were reuniting. I welcomed everyone and we went around the room introducing ourselves.

Ilana spoke about homebirths and birth centers, taking questions as she went along. She blew away some myths with evidence-based research: "Women have *the same* mortality rate at home as low-risk women who birth in hospitals. Homebirth *is* legal. Most catastrophes do *not* happen within minutes. A hospital transfer is always an option," she said. I knew homebirth midwives were CNMs who have the skills and equipment to resuscitate the baby, stop a hemorrhage and help a stalled labor. But she went on to say, "Here, in Israel, the groups of homebirth midwives meet monthly to discuss unusual cases and learn topics of interest. They share information; i.e., new heel pricks for baby and renew skills, i.e., resuscitation."

I was excited about the dynamics and thrilled that the turnout was so successful.

I had a client due that week and was praying she wouldn't call that day. I really did not want to miss this meeting, especially since it was the first. She didn't call! At the end of the morning, I asked for help dividing the responsibilities of money collection, taking notes on the topic being addressed, planning future meetings, and, the most difficult part, informing other professionals. Not everyone had e-mail back then. This part of the organizing I found to be the most frustrating because I took it to heart to notify everyone. When I received some calls the week after saying, "I never heard about the TALI meeting," or "Why couldn't someone call me?" I felt terrible.

After the tedious task of dividing the list of women, with five women volunteering to make four calls each, I thought the weight was off my shoulders. I would "only" have to come up with a speaker and a venue. So, the next speaker was organized, a midwife who taught paramedics at the ambulance service how to assist at emergency homebirths. I sighed with relief. She was going to teach us something we hopefully would never have to use but if we did, we wouldn't be caught off-guard. I was also excited because the midwife was my good friend, Michal, who had her chain snatched years ago when visiting me in Brooklyn. We kept in touch with a yearly call and a couple of letters, but our paths frequently crossed again with she as a midwife, I as a doula.

Then the first call came from one of the volunteers, one day before the meeting. "The phone was busy on and off for three days and then I got no answer." The next call sounded like this: "A child answered, but I left the message anyway. I was too busy to call again to make sure she got the message." The third call sounded like this: "I was away for a few days and called the women when I returned, but only reached two of them."

Everyone's statement was legitimate but the butterflies in my stomach were there, nevertheless. Would there be a respectable turn-out? Would I have enough money to cover the speaker's cost? Would enough women come to justify the effort to organize it? And primarily, would I get a call the next day asking, "Wasn't there supposed to be a meeting this week?"

For the second gathering, twenty women showed up with everyone chipping in an extra five shekels. Good. Speaker's costs were covered. I dreaded the next few days when I knew the calls would come. And, yes, three calls came. "I *really* wanted to hear that talk. I am so disappointed." Or, "My son told me someone called but he wasn't sure what it was about." Okay. I had to come up with a different solution.

The following month's TALI speaker was already organized; an aromatherapist was presenting. The twenty women from the last meeting knew the details. From now on I was going to leave a message on my second phone line and the women would have to be responsible for calling the Sunday/Monday of the week of the meeting to hear the message. Hopefully, this would work. Obviously, this could not be put into practice until after everyone was e-mailed or called for this next meeting.

The next meeting boasted twenty-three doulas. It was a nice-sized gathering, which allowed some newcomers in the field to share their frustration and learn from the seasoned doula's wisdom. The Passover holiday was approaching, which warranted a break. That was really great for me. I appreciated the time off. I hoped we wouldn't lose the momentum.

After Passover we gathered again to be informed about postpartum depression. It was informative, interesting and helped us increase our skills. I had a client who entered into this "black cloud" a year ago, hoping it would never happen again. I picked up on the signs when I called her home one afternoon, 2 weeks after birth, and her husband said, "She is in bed. Hasn't come out yet today." It was noon. "How long has this been going on?" I asked. "A couple of days," he answered. I drove to their house to try to assess the situation and speak to them about post-partum depression. The husband called for professional assistance the next day.

The next meeting had the biggest turn-out ever. There were forty-seven women, not all doulas this time.

Word of mouth brought new participants - childbirth educators and lactation consultants. They had heard that an anesthesiologist was coming with a PowerPoint presentation. They came to hear him. I was excited that the doctor had a great turn-out. It would have been a bit embarrassing for me had a small group appeared. He was extremely busy and was very gracious about coming. He actually was not in favor of anesthesia for birth, but he explained how the process was done, what "cocktails" were used, and statistics on its use as well as harmful side effects. He was balanced, factual, and answered our questions warmly.

Before we knew it, the summer holidays rolled around. We had to wait for the kids to return to school, so our next meeting was held in September. Suddenly, the Jewish New Year was upon us, so until after the High Holidays we were going to break.

As I tried to pick up the momentum again in the late

summer, the same tune re-played itself. More missed phone calls. Others went away and two callers wanted to be replaced. Burnout is what it was called. I was planning my son's Bar Mitzvah. I decided to put TALI on hold. I, for one, had to take care of my family. Someone else would have to take the reins. Besides, there were some other ideas swimming around in my head.

Chapter 12
San Francisco & The Big Plunge

"MY DOULA ONLY met me at the hospital," one caller complained.

"My doctor decided to induce me and my doula had no natural options," another said.

"Do you stay after the birth and visit me at home some time later?"

"Yes, of course."

"Really? I didn't know doulas do that."

Complaints came from moms about what their doulas did that they shouldn't and what they didn't do that they should have done.

"She came to meet me after the induction got hard and a short time before I needed an epidural. There was no advice about any alternatives."

"My doula left me as soon as I got my epidural. I felt so abandoned."

"I learned in my first course that a first birth which was in a breech position had to be a cesarean. My friend told me that she had a doula at her first birth with a private doctor and had a vaginal breech delivery!"

Then I received different types of calls. One woman asked, "Do you train doulas with international certification so they can work in another country?"

A month later another call came from a past client. "Do you give doula courses?"

That's it. I decided to investigate doula training programs. I wanted to create a different type of doula. I also wanted something that would also be recognized internationally, so a woman could move to other countries and still use her training.

Surfing the web, it seemed that my favorite authors and doula "stars" were associated with DONA International. Penny Simkin, Marshall and Phyllis Klaus and others were going to be at the next DONA conference. Reading the requirements I would need to fulfill, I chose DONA as the organization to certify under. I was already a DONA-certified doula so this was the most logical choice. I waited until Moshe returned from work to speak to him about it.

"What do you think?" I said holding onto my seat.

"Do you *really* want to teach?" His green eyes searched my dark brown ones which twinkled as he asked.

"I am a bit nervous about passing the requirements, but I would like to give it a try," I continued.

"You would be a natural. I see how much you want to do this." he said.

"I feel there is a need for this but I never taught before," I answered.

"How much does it cost and what's involved?"

"I would be gone almost two weeks. It's in San Francisco."

I explained the details, money and the certification requirements.

"Go for it," he said with a smile on his face. "I'll hold down the fort." Giving him a peck on the cheek, I couldn't believe what I had just committed to. Searching the DONA International site, I booked the early-bird special to the conference. I chose the workshops I wanted to attend at the conference and signed up for the teacher's workshop.

I would be part of the general sessions absorbing the wisdom of Penny Simkin as she described the physiology of birth through a physiotherapist's viewpoint.

Henci Goer would be there, giving us the latest research and statistics.

I would come back mentally charged and emotionally stimulated while on the road to becoming a doula trainer, too! This was going to be a year of professional growth and challenge.

I then began the search for roommates as I added myself to a list of women looking to share a room. I spoke to a doula friend about coming, who also decided to become a trainer. She and a twenty-year old from somewhere in the States, who was coming as a babysitter, were to be my roommates.

Attending the training was approved, conference paid for, and airline tickets booked. I would cook and freeze main meals for my family, making it a bit easier to cope in my absence.

I was so looking forward to the excitement of a conference that hosted more than 300 women. Certifying meant that I would have mentors to turn to, a magazine with the latest information and being able to continue researching and reading.

The anticipation heightened as the date drew closer. It was July 2003. I bought a new suitcase, packed kosher food, and conferred with my friend to make last-minute arrangements. I also took a small shopping list from the kids.

Landing in San Francisco, a place I hadn't seen since playing tourist twenty years ago, I was captivated. My travel companion didn't share the same enthusiasm. Her children were younger so it was harder to leave, and leaving the Holy Land was not easy. We also had to work around the kosher food issue. We managed to sustain ourselves on tuna, sardines, and the bread we brought with us. We picked up some fruit and delicious crunchy pickles in the local supermarket. Focused on my purpose for being there, food became secondary.

Arriving at the Westin airport hotel gave me a true feeling of vacation. This place would fill my body with much needed rest for a busy mom and working doula; or is that a working mom and a busy doula? The intellectual stimulation would give me the opportunity to return with so much to share with my fellow educators, doulas and especially my future students.

Unlocking the door to our room, I threw myself backwards onto the double-bed feeling like a kid falling onto an inflatable trampoline. I wanted to play as much as to learn. The break from the stress of the everyday routine made me as delirious as the view of the bay from our window.

Thank you, G-d, for this conference. I am ready to meet the stars. Some travel to California to meet movie stars, while I came to meet my birthing stars.

The next five days raced by. Over 300 women poured into the general session which opened the conference.

Educators, doulas, lactation consultants and some midwives networked, while others reunited. The energy was difficult to contain by the time Debra Pascali-Bonero opened the conference presenting her nationwide *"Listening to Mothers"* survey. *That's what it's about*, I thought - listening to mothers. Mothers need to be understood and supported while giving information to make careful decisions. Debra was someone I would enjoy learning from as well as talking to over a cup of tea. Her white smile and blond wavy hair kept me focused while her information expressed through warmth and caring never allowed me to leave my chair.

There were lectures on *Safe and Effective Maternity Care, Induction of Labor, Can Elective Cesareans be Justified* and one of my favorites, *Third Stage of Labor: Why the Panic?*

Of course most of the lectures discussed the doula's role in all this. More focus is now on the doula's role after the birth. With lectures like *Feeding the Postpartum Family* and *Assisting Parents Following the Death of a Stillborn or Premature Baby*, the need for postpartum doulas is growing.

Slide shows, films and Power Points made the topics come alive.

One by one my heroes came to the podium. My favorite authors were fifty feet away. When the break commenced, I had the nerve to follow another woman who asked for pictures together with the stars.

"Do you mind having a picture with me, also?" I feebly asked. I was intimidated by the greatness despite their humbleness.

Dr. Michael Klein and Dr. Harvey Karp, new to me at this time, were part of a breed of doctor we rarely read about. They believed in a woman's ability to give birth and a baby's need for the mom longer than the nine months in-utero.

The break also consisted of filling our tote bags with the latest massage tools and gadgets from the kiosks which lined the walls around the entrance hall. Latest birth books, t-shirts and computer programs to file a doula's information were all there for sale.

Terri Shilling, a captivating teacher whose "Idea Box" would later give me creative tips for teaching was there and so was Kathy McGrath who pops up everywhere. I now use her *"Finding the Path"* tape in my very first class when I am training doulas. She is sensible, understanding and wise. For the doulas reading this book, you know who I am referring to. For the layman reading this book, I do not want to bore you with names of other speakers you don't know.

I wanted to be a doula who incorporates all of their wisdom, talents, skills and energy. I was asking for the impossible. I suppose I will just strive to be the best I can be and leave the rest to G-d.

The end of the conference involved the teacher-training itself. Twelve women from three continents learned from the co-founder herself, Penny Simkin, and her "assistant" Kathy McGrath. We wrote, listened and took different positions on the floor. They made us think. They made us listen. Even more, they gave us a love for learning more and a passion about training doulas.

Chapter 13
An Interview with the Kids

REFLECTING BACK OVER the past few years, while my roommate dozed on the plane, I wondered how my work had been affecting the kids. It didn't seem to matter as much when they were younger because I assumed they became used to it. They didn't have input into my choice of professions. Being a doula was Mom's job.

As my work took me beyond an average doula's practice—lending out birth books, fielding questions from pregnant women who were not my clients, etc.—I decided to have a heartfelt discussion about their feelings. Having started my nightly escapes when my youngest was almost three, I felt like a Clark Kent becoming Superman, especially when a call came and I pulled on my purple lab coat before running off to a birth. I went from baking cookies with the kids and going to PTA meetings to becoming a night owl of sorts. I donned a self-appointed zeal to help save women from a potentially traumatic birth as well as unnecessary interventions. Organizing and attending seminars and conferences had me out of the house frequently. Maybe I was running out too often?

Our home was able to run smoothly while I attended only one or two births a month. Many times I made it home by morning to make sandwiches and kiss the kids good-bye as they boarded the school buses. The prenatal and postpartum meetings could be held when the kids were at school or asleep. The erratic nature of the births was, for my family, most unsettling. After the first couple of years, my monthly clientele began to rise from one per month to as many as four or five!

As word of mouth spread and more calls came in, I saw the house needing more structure. I could freeze dinners ahead of time, but I wasn't always there when my youngest entered the door. Some family appointments I had to postpone and arriving late for PTA meetings became the norm, if I showed up at all! Sometimes I saw the children's sad faces and other times I felt their apathy when I returned home. I would smile saying, "Hi, I am home!" as they would run past me shouting, "Hi Mom. We are going to play!" I didn't want latch-key kids.

I spoke to a neighbor who agreed to watch my three year-old if he arrived home before me or his older siblings. My husband agreed to back me up on those occasional mornings, going to work a bit late so someone would be there to see them off to school. The parenting experts say there are three crucial times of the day when children need their parents: leaving in the morning, returning home, and going to bed at night. Having lived all these years with my schedule, my family had to keep up with my pace.

While attending a birth, I would tell my client I needed the bathroom and would quickly call home. "Good morning. How are you?" I asked whoever answered with much love in my voice. "Are you ready for the bus? So nice that Daddy got you ready. Give him a kiss for me. See you when you come home."

Sometimes I would add, "I am at the hospital near the bakery you like so I will bring you home your favorite cookies. Okay?"

"Sure Mom. Thanks."

One year when the children were older, I decided to hold a family gathering to speak to the kids about my work. It was eight in the evening when even the teens are home (for now). My youngest was already seven, and even he must have known this was not a normal job. He saw his friends' moms home in the evening hours, even if they worked.

"Although you never know when I am coming or going, I am home more than the average nine-to-five working mom," I told them.

"Yeah, Mom, but it is hard not knowing if you are going to be there when we come home. I like to tell you about my day," said my youngest daughter, at nine years old.

"Sometimes I need to talk to you about the guy I am dating," said my eldest.

"You know it helps to bring money into the house so I am hoping we will continue to be in this together," I answered. It was my extra projects that made it more interruptive of our lives. I held my breath for their reactions.

"I'm used to it," said my fourth child, my son who was rarely home anyway.

"This is your work, Mom, and you love it," said my seventeen-year-old daughter. "It's just when you *are* home, you don't have to answer the phone all the time." I thought about this comment later. Just because a phone rang, that didn't mean I *had* to answer it. I had my cell for emergencies.

"I can make our sandwiches in the morning!" said my fourteen-year old. "If you can leave us some food to warm up that would help," said my thirteen-year old son, "so we can help ourselves to food even if you are sleeping."

My eldest, a daughter, now entering college, would have the brunt of the responsibility, but she said she would roll up her sleeves and pitch in. I was so proud of them. I felt a bit guilty that I didn't give them a real choice in the matter but neither did immigrant parents. Of course, in that case it was really a necessity. Was mine? Was a family gathering more of an explanation of what was changing in the routine of our home rather than asking for opinions?

When I grew up, we were always told that a family is not a democracy. As long as the parents agreed, the children would have to follow. One thing I knew: to make this work, we had to keep the children involved in a positive way. How so? Pizza dinners weren't working anymore.

When I arrived home, I would still say with enthusiasm, "Wow, a beautiful baby boy! Healthy and big!" I pulled out some chocolates from the birthing mom saying, "She really appreciated you guys letting me be there. This is her way of saying thank you." Sometimes I actually bought the treats myself.

One day I brought my son a ball and another time I

told my daughter that I was saving up a bit of money from each birth so she could go to summer camp. This way I kept up the family's support of my work.

Things got a bit out of hand when I later opened the lending libraries. Although I made specific hours for my library, some women could not come at those times so they called to come at other times. Being too accommodating, I allowed it, which was often disruptive to the family. I also received phone calls asking, "Where are your libraries located? Can I have the number of the one nearest me?"

When I created a tape of the spirituality of childbirth with a rabbi's wife, I received calls for orders of the tape. So, my home became a Grand Central Station of books, tapes, and information on pregnancy and birth. I had to set borders. Times and days had to be adhered to or my family would not be supportive. How much could I expect of them?

The kids were some of the youngest people I knew with information on birth. When my daughter, who was only nine, once answered the phone whispering, "I think her water broke," I had a good laugh, giving her a hug because I knew she had no idea what that was.

She must have overheard me run out saying to my husband, "Gotta go, her water broke!"

Coming home once, disheartened from a long birth which ended in a cesarean, my eleven-year-old son asked, "What is a cesarean?" I would explain that it is another way for the baby to exit but not the ideal way, feeling that each child should only receive the information they could handle.

A few years later, nine years into my profession, I decided to interview them, each one privately. I asked the same questions regarding my work.

"How did you feel when I ran out to attend a birth, or wasn't home when you woke up or came home from school?"

"What did you tell your friends when they asked you what work your mom did?"

"Would you rather I was a teacher or had another nine-to-five job?"

From my oldest (who was fourteen when I became a doula) to the youngest (who was almost three), the answers went something like this:

Tsippy: "I had to adjust to doing more work when you were sleeping off a birth. Actually, the one time I really didn't like it was when we had a snowstorm in Jerusalem and you were stuck in the hospital. I was busy the whole day changing kids' socks and warming up their gloves so they could go out and get wet all over again. I tried to keep the house from getting soaked, too. It was a big job for a fourteen-year-old."

"Yes it was and you came through with flying colors," I said quietly.

She continued, "I know people appreciate the job you are doing so even though we feel your absence most on the Sabbath, we manage."

My second daughter, Nehama, twenty-one-months younger, only truly appreciated it when she gave birth. "Your knowledge and experience really helped me," she said. "I took your doula course at age twenty-two, but decided it wasn't practical for a young family."

My twenty-one-year-old, practical son Mendy, said, "It's a good job, something you enjoy, you are good to other people and it brings in a good income. The only thing I didn't like was when the house was too pressured and there was no one to help clean or cook. If we had had someone to help us, we would have been calmer." He added, "Teaching would have been less hectic even if you would have been busier."

Mendy was my child who liked change the least. He is structured and disciplined. The sudden rush out the door was not for him. I doubted his wife would be a doula.

My younger ones felt like they were born into this way of life. They were proud of my work, too. I showed them the various letters and notes the birthing women wrote, especially ones that mentioned them. "Your family should be so proud of you. Your self-sacrifice made my birth so wonderful. Thank you." Or another one that said, "Your concern, kindness, and patience (your family's patience too from all my phone calls) made my birth experience so positive."

"We liked the treats and notes you left us on the kitchen table before you went to sleep from an all-night birth. Notes like 'Mazal tov! A cute little boy. Have a nice day,' with little smiley faces on them."

Even though they missed me at certain times, they tried to look at the good side.

"Everybody should take a doula, Mom," announced my teenage daughter."

"I liked running to flag down a cab," said my middle son who enjoys action.

My youngest became an expert at filling up my water bottles that I kept partly frozen until needed. Spreading peanut butter onto my pick-me-up wholewheat crackers and other treats he could do with his eyes closed.

This son, then fourteen years old, said, "I think you should charge more."

"Why?" I asked.

"You are getting old and can't work for too many more years. After that, you can write books. That keeps the memory strong." (I wondered if he was thinking about my mom. He knows Alzheimer's can be hereditary, but this wasn't the time to bring up the subject).

Bless them all. They flowed with me while I pursued my mission while balancing my homemaking. I never envisioned myself as a 24-hour-a-day, stay-at-home mom, but I knew, at least this work made my children proud.

My family, the most important people in my life, understood the truth behind my passion. There was so much work to do. I tried to maintain my equilibrium to be the best doula and mom I could be.

Chapter 14
The World on My Shoulders & Moving Mom to Israel

RECEIVING A CALL one day, almost nine months after we moved mom downtown, Alice said, "Remember you once offered to bring mom to Israel?"

"Yes. I remember," I hesitatingly replied.

"Well, Mom is going to Israel to Nehama's (my daughter) wedding. Why don't you try talking to her about living there?" suggested Alice.

"That won't be easy. She never felt close to Judaism and she was never a Zionist," I answered.

"I know, but we have no choice."

I was speechless. "What's going on?"

"It's gotten really difficult," she continued. "She needs full time care."

"It's come to a point where she needs 24/7 help and it will still be difficult caring for her. Leaving her alone, even part of the day on Sunday, was not possible anymore," she continued. "She left the apartment in the morning and upon returning had to ask the security guard where the elevator was. Then, one Sunday, when alone for a couple of hours, she wandered on the third floor looking for her apartment."

I knew Karen couldn't come on Sundays and the part-time caregivers Alice tried were problematic in many ways. The situation was getting desperate. Alice could not take the strain and the phone calls from that familiar number (Mom's) causing her to run from her job to Mom's apartment to correct an emergency.

That night I shared of the gist of the phone call with Moshe.

"Maybe we should seriously think about moving mom to Israel."

"We will have to check out rental apartments and old age homes and see what our options are," he replied.

"We also have to know what she is eligible for as a new immigrant."

"I know," I said nervously. "Medical coverage could be an obstacle since she has a pre-existing condition.

"You know this will probably be a permanent move even though we are going to just try it out," I stated.

What a guy, I thought. *This won't be easy.*

Deep inside, we both knew this would be a final decision.

Our lives would be in an upheaval with another dependent, but I only have *one* mom. I was nervous but certain about what had to be done.

Losing a job is disappointing, sometimes debilitating. Losing a limb is a horrible major adjustment. But losing one's mind is frightening beyond belief. It means loss of words, memories and one's entire essence. Other than medication to slow it down, there is nothing to be done. There is a loss of control as the plaques form in the brain. The race against time to find a cure is happening worldwide. But for now, we had to seriously think about moving mom once again, this time to Israel.

A few days later, and after much research and many conversations, Moshe and I decided that immigrating was our mother's only option. It was a major change, true, but here she would have a daughter, son-in-law and six children to share the responsibility with a caregiver. It had to be the best solution—it was the *only* solution.

Alice went to the aliyah department in Philadelphia to find out what she needed to do from there. So, less than three months before my daughter's wedding, my days and my dreams were filled with greater anxiety than the norm. My 19-year-old bride was also extremely busy with school, tests and wedding plans. I ran to Mom in America, ran to the wedding hall when back in Israel, searched desperately for the right apartment for my mom, wrote an invitation list, interviewed caregivers, looked for wedding clothes, took care of the bureaucratic logistics of Mom's immigration, helped to hire a photographer, band and arrange short term rental apartments for the groom's family to stay in. I had to juggle these myriad responsibilities, including making peace between everyone, while keeping myself from sinking! Moshe did more than his share of running too.

Would the new in-laws, coming from out of the country, be happy with the apartment we rented for them? Would my sisters be happy with the apartment I found for my Mom? Some places had been a third floor walk-up; others were dark, while others too small. This was just right, but how would they know? I was frantically trying to please everyone, including my twelve-year-old daughter, who wanted the perfect dress for her sister's wedding. We ran out of time, so she settled for something else. I was so happy when she received loads of compliments.

I flew to the States to bring my Mom over one month before the wedding. The beginning took adjustment. After all, there was a new apartment and a lovely caregiver from the Philippines named Lydia. Mom was only a five- minute walk away so I visited every day and she visited me. We played Scrabble which she begged me to play, despite her frustration. She couldn't even think of even three letter words and, when she did, even those were spelled wrong. Once she threw the board out of anger and frustration. I cried and held her tightly. "I love you, Mom," I said. Then I added "I am so sorry. So, so, sorry."

We all danced at the wedding, the in-laws were fine with their apartment, and Mom's place was light and airy so everyone liked it. There were a few criticisms about the furniture but moving hers to Israel would have been logistically difficult. "We can always change the sofa if it doesn't work out," I told them. Slowly, as the guests returned to their respective countries, life began to return to normal.

Emerged in the world of birthing, and studying for my degree as a doula trainer, coupled with Mom right nearby, "normal" took on a different meaning.

Chapter 15
The Wheelchair Birth

"HI, SARAH!" BEGAN the hysterical call from my good friend, Amy. "I got to week 38 but my out-of-control eating habits have sent my blood pressure out of control. They decided to induce labor and although you warned me, I am not prepared for this."

"I am sorry. I know what a busy mother of eight you are, but we women must find the time to take care of ourselves."

"I know. I know. Now the new school year is starting in exactly one week. My blood pressure had always been a little high - did it have to shoot up now, with September 1st only one week away? There are still books to buy, skirts to hem and shoes to get. The children were supposed to be well into a schedule when this baby was born."

"Okay. Take a deep breath and tell me how I can help. Let's deal with the situation you are in and forget the 'could have, should haves'."

"On Tuesday evening they were going to give me that Pitocin drug to get the labor going, but the baby was still high in the uterus and apparently not quite ready. The doctor decided to wait and watch. Instead, I was to have hospital bed rest."

"For how long?" I asked.

"Until Saturday night and then we will see," was the reply.

"There is not a lot you can do now. Trust their judgment and wait it out. Maybe a reflexology treatment will help get your body naturally prepared for labor. I will try to get hold of someone. Meantime, ask your doctor."

Amy was put on blood pressure medication, which helped the first day before it rose again. Seeing it was beginning to peak, they sent her for some tests, including an ultrasound. "Whatever you need to do, just do it. In any case, I can't get hold of a reflexologist during summer vacation. This was just a potential help. You are really high-risk now. You know this can be very dangerous for the baby, too. Just give birth already."

The next morning Amy called. This was her story of "divine providence."

Finding the ultrasound room was no easy task. She was in a major Jerusalem hospital, and the room was located at the far end. She had to make her way down long passageways with the lights dimmed at that late hour. It was quite unnerving, but she had to go.

She decided not to call her husband since he had his hands full as it was. An ultrasound was a fairly simple procedure. If they decided to proceed with any intervention, she would call him to come.

Throughout the days she had to be in the hospital she kept repeating in her mind, *I will be home on Tuesday when school starts. My kids are not going to start their first day of school without me!* Everyone thought she was crazy. She would have to give birth by the next morning, Sunday, to be out by Tuesday, and she was far from giving birth.

Finally she arrived at the ultrasound room, only to find it locked. Amy was distracted by the sound of someone crying. She spotted a woman sitting in a wheelchair, apparently waiting for the ultrasound technician to arrive. She was there because her labor was not progressing. They suspected that the umbilical cord was wrapped around the baby's body, holding it back from coming out. They had sent her for an ultrasound to see if this was the cause. Whoever had wheeled her there had left her alone so she could take care of something (hopefully to find the technician). The woman had thrombosis so she was sitting with her leg bandaged. There was no possibility for her, in that condition and at her weight (almost twice my size), to wheel herself to find help.

As her contractions strengthened and came closer, Amy realized there was only one thing to do. "Let's go," she said courageously. Amy pushed her down those long corridors, trying to remember the way back to the delivery rooms, forgetting about her high blood pressure problem. Suddenly Amy felt contractions: *I am in labor*, she thought!

The woman's contractions were coming so fast that she was concentrating on finding her way back as quickly as possible. When they arrived, huffing, at the delivery rooms, the sight must have been amazing—Amy, with her large-proportioned body, pushing her companion, almost double her size, with Amy screaming, "She's about to give birth!"

Seeing her pushing, the midwives tilted the chair

backward, put on their gloves and, with Amy still holding the wheelchair, her new friend gave birth.

Thanks to her, and the exertion of pushing the wheelchair to the other end of the hospital, Amy gave birth forty-five minutes later!

P.S. She was always grateful to Amy, and they've been close for over ten years!

Chapter 16
Staff Relations & Finding Common Ground

TO CONNECT OR bond with the hospital staff was a topic addressed by Penny Simkin in the DONA conference. I bought a CD called *"Communicating with Hospital Staff"*. Brenda Lane spoke about *"Communicating with Challenging People,"* our family members and even our clients sometimes! In years to come, I would give out this CD to my future doula students.

With most women giving birth in a hospital setting, it is imperative that we doulas learn to navigate the system. Many of us have a world view of birth which tends to lean towards the natural birth experience while working within a system of protocols and lawsuits. If something "happens", a hospital can get sued. So can the doctor as well as the midwife. As non-medical personnel, doulas do not have the pressure of a lawsuit hanging over their heads. Although we may know, for instance, that research shows the EFM (electric fetal monitor) does not improve outcomes, hospital staff is dependent on it for their defense in a potential lawsuit. While we believe in *intermittent* monitoring, we can advocate for it by showing our clients the research. In the meantime, we can at least request that the laboring woman be allowed to stand with the monitor. If the fetal heart rate is fine, why not stand? I know the staff learned to strap on the belts while she lies down, but it makes birth so much more painful. So I say to my clients, "Ask to stand up if that's what feels right to you." I want to work as a team rather than "us" vs. "them."

Entering a hi-tech hospital that was undergoing a metamorphosis towards a more natural birth environment, my client was in very active labor. Susan was having her sixth baby. Five centimeters open with contractions every four minutes, she entered the delivery room heading straight for the shower.

"Susan, this is Aviva. She will be your midwife."

"Hi there. I really need a shower now. Is it okay?"

"As long as the baby was monitored in the receiving (triage) room, no problem."

"Hello, Aviva. Haven't seen you in a few weeks." Aviva, who was usually very pleasant, had a different look on her face. Greeting me with a nod was not her style. Her energy was low and her eyes did not exude their usual warmth.

"Is everything alright? You seem to look sad today." Although I had worked with her only a few times, we had a pleasant working relationship. Yet we knew nothing about each other's personal lives except that we lived one neighborhood from the other.

"Well, yes."

"Do you want to talk about it?" I asked.

"My daughter is in a hospital being treated." I was surprised at her forthrightness. It seemed she needed to share and I was willing to listen.

"How old is she, what happened?" I patiently asked while Susan is showering.

"She's my seventeen-year-old. Has anorexia. She's in a hospital program to treat it," she explained. The pain of her daughter's ordeal was clearly seen through her dark brown eyes.

"I am so sorry." I was caught off guard. Who would have expected her to share *that?* I had read about anorexia and bulimia but never encountered someone who suffered from it. There was talk in my high school about a skinny girl in another class who had an eating disorder. Now it seemed more exposed and talked about. Certainly Aviva seemed like a nice down-to-earth mom with no pretenses or issues, or problems in her life.

I took her hand and held it warmly as she smiled and said thank you.

"How much longer does she have to stay there?"

"Hard to say. It may take one more month in the hospital followed by an outpatient program."

"Can I give you a hug? I am a mother, too. This must be so hard to take."

Aviva returned my embrace as only one mother to another can.

"I really wish you lots of inner strength. G-d bless both of you."

Aviva began to sort through Susan's paperwork. I made myself busy removing some tools from my bag of tricks. Knocking lightly on the bathroom door, I asked Susan how she was.

"All's fine. I like your new green music CD."

Aviva, eyeing my latest blue and white massage tool, asked, "What is that?"

The eight, tiny tractor tires roll as I guide the arched

handle across a woman's lower back. "Turn around," I said to Aviva. Running the tool up and down her back, I asked, "How does this feel?"

"Great. I am ready to have another baby," she answered with a smile, both of us knowing the "factory" was no longer in operation.

I continued for a few minutes until it was time for Susan's baby to be monitored.

Susan came out of the shower to be checked.

"Eight centimeters!" Aviva said as she turned to open the delivery kit.

"Can I stand now with the monitor?" Susan asked.

"As long as the heartbeat reads out okay," Aviva answered. "But let me know if you feel pressure."

"No problem. Thanks so much".

Forty-five minutes later, Susan felt pressure. Upon examination, Aviva said she could begin pushing.

"Mazal tov! Here is your baby girl." I wondered if Aviva had flashbacks into birthing her own daughter and thinking about what her sweet baby is doing now, hoping she will become well. After Aviva assisted with the delivery of the placenta she then supported Susan to nurse her baby girl. I usually take this role; however, Aviva seemed to want more involvement.

After letting the parents bond, Aviva and I step out of the room. I handed her a present, a box of After Eight dinner mints. "Thanks. You didn't have to."

"I know but you work hard, so why not?"

Before going home, I looked into Aviva's eyes, saying a slow farewell.

On my way out of the delivery rooms, I saw men pacing, some leaning against a wall sleeping upright, and an ambulance driver wheeling in a woman in a panic as she was ready to deliver. In a hospital which boasted over 1,000 births a month, the midwives would be having a busy night. It must be difficult sometimes to emotionally give when a midwife is physically or emotionally exhausted. We doulas can help foster a relationship between staff and clients by encouraging our clients to write thank-you notes, bring a present and give the staff the respect they deserve.

Chapter 17
More Staff Relations

A FEW MONTHS later, I had registered for an evening lecture about Alzheimer's. I was so excited to see a familiar ob/gyn at an Alzheimer's conference. This was another opportunity to connect with staff, although I kept in mind that not everyone would be interested in "connecting."

Making eye contact with the doctor, I walked in his direction. The room was subdued as people headed toward the coffee table to chat with the speakers or each other. Maybe it was the topic at hand or the late hour. Giving a nod, I asked the doctor, "Are you here for a family member?"

"Yes, my father."

"Is he still at home?" I inquired.

"Yes, but we may have to find him a facility in a few months. And you?"

"My mom. She is eight years into this awful disease. We moved her to Israel almost a year ago. She is still in a rented apartment near me with her caregiver. We have to move her soon. She isn't steady on her feet; soon she'll need a wheelchair."

"Good luck with her," he closed the conversation with a warm smile.

"Also to you, with your dad."

Staff members have personal issues and problems to handle. They are people, too. I try to remember this even in the heat of a labor when we may not agree how to handle the situation. Although we don't have to agree with everything they advise, we have to have dialogue and not go into the hospital with boxing gloves on. Assertive? Sometimes. Aggressive? Never. Working as an informed team will get us a much more positive and safe birth experience for our clients.

I was in a fun mood one day on my way to a birth. I had just bought a battery-operated massager which was going to be put to use. Packing three spare batteries into my birth bag, I smiled wondering what took me so long to buy a bag on wheels. I call it my "bag of tricks".

In my early doula days it was light-filled with two aromatherapy oils of peppermint and organic orange, a hot water bottle, relaxation music with a small cassette recorder and a washcloth.

As years went by, the conferences I attended and books I read gave me ideas about adding more options. I ordered "green" (nature sounds) relaxation music, a Rebozo scarf, a cutting board for extra back pressure, baby hats with pink and blue stripes, an instruction paper for early nursing tips, ice packs, spray bottles for the mother's hair and face (especially in transition) and a bottle of castor oil in case she needs help getting the contractions going.

"You making a salad after the birth?" asked a midwife seeing the cutting board.

"I am taking this room!" said the midwife coming on

shift, hearing her favorite classical music coming from my portable speakers.

Walking into the hospital with my carry-on suitcase made staff smile, and a few asked, "When is your flight?"

It's true. I looked as if I was getting ready to board a plane. "As soon as this birth is over, I hope!"

This third birth progressed quickly, but in the process I took out my new battery massager. How it helps to make the atmosphere even more positive and upbeat than it is! It is downright friendly! Finishing within two hours of arrival, the midwife was interested in trying it. I massaged her back while mom was nursing. She really enjoyed it. "You midwives work really hard. You should keep one of these handy for each other."

Naomi called in another midwife to show her and I massaged her back, too. Another two midwives came over when they saw something was happening in room number ten. It became a party atmosphere. Naomi asked, "Where did you buy this?"

"One of the shops in the central bus station," I answered.

"I never get there. Can you pick one up for me?"

"No problem," I answered, not knowing the next time *I* would be there. "It may take me a week or two."

"Doesn't matter," she answered after handing me 100 shekels.

When I bring items to share with my birthing mom, I try to include the midwife so she doesn't feel left out. I ask her if she would like to smell the aromatherapy oils and ask the staff to take some cookies and chocolates. "Here, this will help you get through the night shift."

Many times I bring them something totally separate, just for them, to show my appreciation. A hand cream or a pretty coffee mug filled with sweets goes a long way.

Jokes also can pick up the mood, especially if the staff are busy or tired.

Depending on the person, I take the liberty to make personal jokes, but I am careful to remember my role there.

Once, a doctor said to the midwife and me, "Look at this great stitch job." (It was from a small tear). "Not bad, if I say so myself."

I responded, "When you get tired of this shift work, you can become a tailor!" We all had a laugh.

Working with doctors can bring us to a humbling place many times. I have to give credit where credit is due. Doctors go through ten years of college, medical school, residency/internship, at the expense of a social life, sufficient sleep and family life. Residents and interns work twenty or more grueling hours at a time, ending in exhaustion with nutritionless, eat on the run food. I have seen the man or woman in greens looking as if they have been through a war zone - bloodshot eyes, wrinkled brow, and slumped shoulders. I've wondered if they were training for endurance in case of the next war.

So, when I encounter a doctor, tired or not, resident or not, I always smile. If they do not acknowledge my presence, I at least nod my head. One never knows when we may find ourselves working in the same room together. We certainly want to be able to co-exist, even if our perspectives are a bit different. Most importantly, we both want a healthy mom and healthy baby. However, the process and the definition of "healthy" can be dissimilar. For example, an induction with Pitocin followed by an epidural may be the doctor's framework of a normal, healthy birth process, and mine may be to wait and see if she enters labor naturally. If not, there is acupuncture, castor oil, and a host of other, safer methods.

When my client, Rebecca decided to hire Dr. Baron, I was thrilled – and not because the midwives don't know how to help a woman deliver her baby. Many of these caregivers have assisted at hundreds, if not thousands, of births. I was thrilled because Dr. Baron is "cool". I haven't used that word in over thirty-five years. He is one of the most chilled-out, but experienced, doctors I know. He works at a hi-tech medical center in Jerusalem, but he is as low-tech as they come.

The day arrived and Rebecca began labor, her first, with the traditional, expected pattern. "They began a couple of hours ago," she explained in the mid-morning phone call.

"They are about ten minutes apart, lasting thirty seconds."

"Sounds normal," I replied. "You may want to nap so you will have strength when it picks up. Call me later."

Six hours later, with a hearty vegetable soup coming to a boil, the phone rang again. "Hi. It's Rebecca." We had a chat about the contractions getting closer and stronger. She told me she's managing well.

"Let me help you breathe through the next couple of

contractions while I time them. Do you want to have a warm shower while I serve dinner? I will come right after. But Rebecca, if you need me sooner, phone right away. Oh, and try to eat something light and easy to digest. Some pasta or fruit would be good."

"That's fine. Come right after dinner," she chirped, sounding too good to be in active labor.

After serving dinner, I packed up a thermos full of soup, a healthy dinner for a woman after birth.

Arriving an hour later, I found Rebecca in the shower, having been in there for twenty minutes. "Hi there!" I hollered so she could hear me above the shower's roar. "There are some strong ones, but mostly they are doable," she answered from behind the red-flowered shower curtain. "You can come in."

"About how often are they coming?" I quieted down to keep the mood calm.

"Still about five-six minutes apart."

"Want to come out of the shower for a change of pace?" Rebecca agreed. The bathroom felt claustrophobic and had gotten very steamy. "I want a ten-minute break," pleaded Rebecca. "I'm sure you do," I replied. I put on waterfall relaxation music, dimmed the lights, and brought out the aromatherapy oils. Smelling a few different types, she decided on the lavender. We continued with a massage, only pausing for Rebecca to get on her hands and knees to sway with every contraction. I pressed on her back to relieve the pain.

Making sure her husband felt involved, I asked him to fill up the hot water bottle. "Do you want to eat something? It could be a long night," I whispered to him, not wanting to discourage his wife. "It's a good idea to pack some food for the hospital too."

"When will we be going?" David asked.

"Depends on the two of you. In her birth plan, Rebecca wanted to stay home as long as possible."

I suggested they call Dr. Baron. "It's a good idea to ask if we can stay home longer and it would be nice to give him a heads-up so he can make his evening plans."

David called and announced, "We can stay longer, but when they reach about three-minute intervals or if the water breaks, we should come in."

"Great," responded Rebecca. "I am just not ready to leave my bedroom."

Pity Dr. Baron doesn't attend home births, I thought. *We are only ten minutes from the hospital if we would need to transfer.*

Two hours later we were on our way with contractions three-minutes apart.

"Hello, Dr. Baron."

"Rebecca, how are you?"

"It's really getting hard."

"Let's check to see how you are progressing. First births can take awhile."

He is always so positive.

"Completely effaced and four centimeters!" he announced.

We really wanted to hear more.

"Great," he continued. "You are in good, active labor."

Still not wanting to take pain meds, Rebecca decided another shower may help her. She also chose to take an enema even though it is not required these days. She was told it could help bring the head down.

It's now well past midnight, as the ticking of the clock was overpowered by the monitor registering the baby's heartbeat and the strength of Rebecca's contractions. Dilation had not progressed. I had Rebecca try side lunges; a semi-plie for those ballerinas out there. I used the Rebozo (Mexican shawl) technique to help change the baby's position and *anything* to help labor to progress, but nothing was helping.

With a heavy heart, Rebecca agreed on the Pitocin, the synthetic form of the body's oxytocin which helps increase contractions to speed up labor. After two hours of slowly raised Pitocin and one centimeter progression, her yawns and tears told it all. She was spent, emotionally and physically. Rebecca opted for an epidural.

The epidural helped Rebecca relax but after some time, the Pitocin was shut off due to decelerations in the baby's heartbeat. The heartbeat returned quickly, so Dr. Baron waited to take further action.

As I got nervous and tired, I wondered if her dilation of six centimeters was enough to wait. Was it worth doing a c-section now while the baby was still okay? Why should we wait until there was a serious problem? What was happening to me? *Of course it is not worth doing a cesarean now! She will be considered high risk forever!!* I learned all the drawbacks and potential problems for future pregnancies and births. No one was even mentioning a c-section, not even her doctor. But mom, baby, and even the doula were very tired. Should I call in a back-up at this hour? My judgment was compromised. I decided to wait it out a bit longer.

We changed Rebecca's position again, laying her on her left side. Dr. Baron started the Pitocin again, watching the baby's reaction carefully. All was okay for a while. After an hour she progressed to seven centimeters, but even after giving Rebecca oxygen, he had to shut off the Pitocin again. There were some more decelerations in the baby's heartbeat but slight ones. Focusing on the ticking of the clock and the heartbeat from the monitor, I was starting to lose faith. Following Dr. Baron out of the room I asked him, "Are you thinking about a cesarean? He said to me, with a colleague of his standing next to us, "The *doula* asks if *I* am thinking about a cesarean and the doctor says, 'No reason we can't wait'." We all had a good laugh and I sent David out to get me a soda from the machine. By 7:30 a.m., Rebecca had a vaginal delivery. She gave birth to an eight-pound baby boy with his hand by his head, probably having slowed the progression of labor. I think I needed a day away from birthing.

Chapter 18
The First Getaway

FEELINGS OF EMOTIONAL and physical exhaustion can overwhelm the most dedicated professional. Calling my good friend, a doula herself, I said, "Everyone needs a vacation, especially a doula. No?"

"Especially you," she responded. "You go beyond the basic doula's work."

Water, whether ocean or a lake, is my favorite place to unwind. A vast blue ocean with wave crests bellowing in and out while the warmth of the orange sun sets, allow me to regain focus while recharging my batteries.

An escape is a simple way of running down the road called "life" without tripping over our own feet. There are the phone calls the doula receives from strangers who need information and emotional support, or the interrupted night's sleep while a woman breathes through a contraction asking her doula to come. There are the emotional highs of a successful VBAC birth and the heart-breaking lows of a lost baby. Even the most normal nine-to-five jobs get a day off or take a sick day. Then there are the two-week (or more) vacations a year giving one the renewed energy to rededicate oneself to the job.

We independent workers have to schedule our own vacations. Most jobs have busy seasons when it is impossible to lose work time. My brother-in-law, a landscaper, can only go on vacation after a long spring, summer and fall of planting and lawn-designing. Accountants can't be reached until way past April 15th and store owners have end-of-the-year stock taking.

Doulas are always on call. Babies have no season, especially when the clients are Orthodox Jews, who have no reason to schedule pregnancies. When babies come, we welcome them. The excitement of never knowing when the phone will ring can be overshadowed by what we call burnout. At some point, we have to be told, "Take a vacation." If our inner voice doesn't tell us, then our children or husbands probably will.

"Mom, you are grumpy a lot."

"Sweetie, you really have bags under your eyes."

"Mom, you haven't read us a bedtime story in two weeks."

"Honey, you okay?"

Picking up the phone, I called my favorite spa at the Dead Sea. "Is there a place for a massage tomorrow at 9:30 a.m?" The smelly sulphur pools and the calm of the Dead Sea were calling me. It is a place where I can sit under the whirlpool baths by my anonymous self - sans cell phone. Thank G-d they haven't yet invented a waterproof cell phone. The salty beach with separate men-women solariums will allow the sun to bake my muscles, tiring me out just enough to fall asleep under the shade of a palm tree.

I am blessed that we live only a one-hour's drive away. Deciding that Moshe could also use a change of scenery, I insisted he come with me.

His sedentary, home-based translation and editing job, staring at a computer screen, also needed to be altered so the stiffness and carpal tunnel don't set in. Agreeing to come, I warmly thanked him. He is as driven as I am with work, community projects and time for prayers and daily Torah learning, as well as child rearing.

The sun rises early in the summer, and the grocery store opens at 7:00, which gave me time to run to buy a few more things. Leaving the sleeping children to "sleep in" during their end-of the year vacation, I wrote an "I love you" note, laying it on the kitchen table with some treats. We had told them we would be going.

Turning the key in our Renault 19 at 8:00 a.m., we were on our way. Bathing suits and multi-colored beach towels were packed with some granola bars, frozen water and orange juice bottles. We were going to experience a cleansing; a true physical and mental get-away.

It was a crystal clear sky, the usual for summer and fall weather in a country where it doesn't rain from May until October or November. The predicted temperature was 85F (29.4 C) degrees. By late morning, right after my massage, we would be under the palm trees and out of the solarium.

Riding down the newly paved road, ready for the tourist season, we wound our way from the Jerusalem hilltops turning toward the sandy slopes which would lead us towards our oasis in the desert. Enjoying the speckled landscape of brush and cactus, I popped some music into the CD player. No homes, no buildings, no sirens from ambulances or police cars. My children were instructed to call only in case of emergency. My cell phone was off. I would check for messages every hour.

After parking the car, Moshe carried the red and white cooler bag, I the canvas tote with the rest of our gear. We looked and felt like tourists. Fifteen minutes to go until my massage, I decided to browse in the gift shop. "What interests you?" asked Moshe. "My treat."

Looking around, I spotted some Dead Sea hand cream. Waving it in the air I said, "This is always good for the lady who washes her hands a lot, mom or doula, and I am both." Removing his wallet from his pocket, he paid for the cream.

"Maybe I should buy extra as presents for the midwives?"

Will my mind ever not wander to the birthing rooms?

The day was spectacular. The massage relaxed me and the sun baked deeply into my muscles, tanning me with a healthy color that would allow me to avoid make-up for at least a week. "Did you learn a new massage technique for your clients?" Moshe asked.

"You know, I really wasn't thinking about my clients."

"Oh really?" he responded with a smile.

"Sure you don't want a massage?" I asked him.

"No. You know I am not into massage."

I checked the cell-phone- no calls. Heading inside to the mineral pools, we sat in the "his and her" pools, relaxing as the Jacuzzi allowed the water to circulate.

Now it was time to return outside to rest under the palm trees. Amazing how they stay luxurious year-round. Lying under a tree, I slept for over an hour. Awakening to see Moshe munching on some granola bars and sipping orange juice, I joined him. "We're returning to the sixties granola generation." I told him. We cracked some jokes, relaxed and spoke for two hours uninterrupted.

To be honest, I had put the latest DONA International magazine in my handbag. I controlled my obsessive behavior by allowing myself to read one article. Like I always say, if I have to be obsessive with something, better birth than some other vice. Deciding it was time to head home, we packed up and walked towards the car.

Making our way back up the road with barely a car passing us by, the mango glow of the sun was lowering over the horizon. I was ready to face a new day, which, for a doula, sometimes begins at night.

With a full night's sleep after a beautiful day's vacation, the phone rang at 5:00 the next afternoon. Yes, it was a woman in labor. Didn't sound like a false alarm.

When I am helping a woman find her own inner strength as she brings forth life into the world, I sometimes have to wear a mask of strength, courage and energy. Some days it is thin or non-existent. I am right there with her; breathing, swaying, massaging. But there are times that the mask is a bit thicker and I pray she won't see I am not really there. Oh, physically I am doing everything she needs to help her birth progress naturally. Emotionally, I am somewhere else. Maybe I am thinking about my best friend having her first daughter's engagement party. I really wanted to be there. Okay, I will bring a back-up to the birth for the wedding itself, but I also wanted to be in her home that night. I already have a daughter married and I wanted to share all these special moments in life with my friend. There are just *so* many reasons I can bring in a substitute. An engagement party is not one of them, especially if it isn't my own daughter's. This I could not justify. Now, the missed evening has schlepped into the wee hours of the morning and I am tired.

"You are doing so well, keep going," even at midnight. *What I really want to be doing is hugging my pillow and snuggling under my comforter. I haven't had much sleep this week; one child was sick, another had a late night graduation. The getaway made this birth doable. I have to be strong.*

"Six centimeters! Not much longer now. It can really pick up and go fast." *I do want her to finish. I want to go home.*

"Let's move some more. How about another shower? You enjoyed it in there before."

I gave her a drink and took one for myself. I smiled, a sincere smile, despite the tiredness behind it.

As she was showering, I closed my eyes thinking, *"Don't look too tired. Her husband may see. I don't want him to feel bad."*

"Are you doing OK in there?"

"Fine," was her reply. I heard it getting harder.

"Do you want to come out or should I come in to help?"

As I went in, I prayed *"G-d, please give me the strength to keep going."*

When my eyes blinked from tiredness she noticed. "You're tired aren't you?" she asked.

"A bit. But I am getting a second wind." *I'm lying. I am trying to get a second wind. Thank G-d she is ten centimeters.* There was a lull between the final pushes and suddenly a cry, a cry of a baby filling his lungs with air for the first time.

Staying only a half an hour after the birth, I asked permission to go. Usually I stay at least an hour to help with the initial breastfeeding, give her a warm drink, and support her with suturing, when needed. Judy was a "seasoned" mom so she didn't need me.

Getting in the taxi, I closed my eyes, leaned against the back of the seat with my arms dropping beside me, envisioning my pillow.

"Bed, here I come."

Chapter 19
The 16th Birth

"SARAH, I NEED your help with a very special pregnant woman," said the familiar voice at the other end of the line, a doula named Libi. She continued, "This is her sixteenth baby, bless her. Are you still there?"

"Yes. Tell me more."

"I received a phone call from a woman who is due this week. She only recently heard about this idea of having a doula" Her name is Chaya. She is a very modest, ultra-Orthodox woman and prefers to have someone from outside of her community. She feels more comfortable having someone help her whom she isn't likely to see again."

"Tell me more about her."

"All fifteen of her previous births were with pain medication, usually Demerol. Her memory of her births is just a blur. She wants to *be* there this time."

"How brave of her."

"She has a friend that hired me for her eighth birth. This friend really inspired her that it was possible to have a wonderful, non-medicated birth! She really encouraged her and now she wants to try!"

"I was with her friend but, again, Chaya wants someone anonymous.

"If you are interested, you need to know that she will also need a significant discount. They really don't have the means to cover the regular cost of a doula." Libi concluded.

"What a privilege," I responded excitedly! "If she has a wonderful birth, she may inspire all her sisters, daughters, cousins, aunts and nieces! What a wonderful opportunity to start a positive ripple effect in her community. Of course I will attend this birth!"

Chaya called me later that day and we set up our first tentative meeting for Wednesday morning at a local coffee shop.

Instead, we met at the hospital! When she called me, she suspected that her waters had broken. Labor had already started.

"I went to the hospital last night when the contractions were irregular," Chaya explained to me at 7:30 a.m. "I was sure my waters broke, but apparently they didn't!"

"Why are you still there now?" I asked.

"They decided if I was already here, they would monitor the baby and see if labor would pick up."

"Are you making nice progress?" I asked.

"I am 90% effaced and two centimeters. It is getting a bit harder so I may need you soon."

"No problem," I told her. "I'll jump in the shower now. I can arrive within the hour!"

"Two centimeters?" I wondered whether or not she should even remain in the hospital. (hmmm)

When I arrived at the hospital, I met Chaya for the first time. She was a smiling, "older" woman wearing a navy head scarf. She reminded me of the grandmother I never had but would have wanted. Three of my grandparents died before I was born, and my only grandma lived in New York, which was too far from Philadelphia for us to see her enough to develop a close relationship. By the time I was a teen she developed cancer, and died. Chaya seemed the type to knit booties and hold the grandchildren for burping on her broad shoulders. I warmly smiled as I approached her. She was a large women and I knew I would have to do my best to massage her in a strong, effective way. I wanted, like with every woman I accompany, to give her my best. Despite that this was her sixteenth time giving birth, the only way she would progress (as in previous births) was with the assistance of some slowly introduced Pitocin drip.

One doctor had recommended a cesarean a few hours earlier. He was afraid of uterine rupture in a "multipara"- a woman who has had so many births before. She did not understand why she was at risk any more than previous times, so she had refused.

By the time I arrived, Chaya was three centimeters. There was time for us to get acquainted, so we enjoyed the chance to exchange more background information about each other.

I told her about my six children and my work as a doula for the past six years. I spoke about my life in Safed before moving to Jerusalem.

"How about you? Tell me something about yourself," I said.

"I have fifteen children and eight grandchildren, thank G-d."

I realized this child would have nephews and nieces ten years *older* than him or /her. How neat!

"Yiddish is my first language. Do you speak Yiddish at all?" she asked.

"No, but my great grandparents surely did!"

We conversed in our common language, Hebrew. She was wearing black and navy attire, while I wore my favorite purples and pinks. Though our background and upbringing were culturally very different, here we were together, sharing an intimate bonding experience.

Then her contractions started to pick up. Only we two were in the room, while her equally quiet and modest husband stood just outside in the hallway, behind the curtain, praying for her to have an easy, safe birth. I saw his sidelocks and long black frock swaying as he prayed.

Chaya was content that her husband was nearby but not in the room. Her mother had helped her through many of her earlier births. They both felt birth was an arena for women.

I spoke in a soothing voice as we made a lot of eye contact. Chaya was able to go inside herself and focus as her contractions became more intense.

"Hot water bottle?" I asked as I lay it gently on her back.

"That feels so good," she said, closing her eyes leaning her head back on the pillow.

We said psalms together in between contractions.

Chaya was in good spirits, feeling grateful to the One who had blessed her with another baby, who she hoped would soon be in her arms.

"Chaya, if there is *anything* you need or want, please tell me. We didn't have a chance to discuss your birth or how I could help you." I said.

"Would you like a sip of water?" I asked.

"That would be nice," she responded.

"There is an ice machine if you would like it colder?"

"I will try it colder. I am getting very warm," she said.

Reaching in my bag, I removed a new washcloth that says *Mazal Tov* on it. I use them to wipe a brow in transition, giving it as a keepsake after the birth.

Two hours passed quickly, when Chaya declared, "Pressure. I am beginning to feel pressure,"

I pressed the nurse's call button.

The midwife, who had just checked Chaya ten minutes earlier, returned promptly to our room saying, "I'm not checking her again. She was only three or four centimeters! Call me again if she really feels like she needs to push," she said as she shut off the IVAC, the machine administering the slow drip of Pitocin that they had started two hours earlier. She smiled pleasantly as she left the room.

Three minutes later Chaya screamed, "The baby's coming!"

I quickly told her husband that he should try to get the midwife to come back.

Then I turned to Chaya, saying calmly with a smile, "Don't worry. At worst, the baby will come out onto the bed. With barely one push, Chaya's beautiful newborn baby girl slipped easily onto the bed.

Then the midwife arrived to be greeted by the sight of a stunned, ecstatic, newly empowered mom.

"I told you the baby was coming," said Chaya. "I finally birthed my own baby!"

Chapter 20
Blue Skies Turn Gray

SOMETIMES IT ISN'T smooth sailing. Skies aren't so blue and the cumulus clouds can turn grey and angry. Then I figure that a doula has done something dumb. It isn't that we are beyond reproach. We aren't perfect. There are times when a doula feels so close to the birthing mom that we speak for her instead of letting her speak. "She doesn't want an epidural."

We take liberties that we shouldn't. "If it hurts so much to be monitored in bed, so stand up with the monitor." We *should* run it past the midwife.

The relationship can be one of support, but sometimes it turns to one of over-dependence. I, personally, am thrilled when I run into one of my previous birthing moms with her new baby and she says, "I had this baby by myself! I did the movements you showed me, waited at home till the contractions became strong, and arrived at eight centimeters." I am so proud. If all my clients continued to take me to assist them at subsequent births, I would never see my family, attend a wedding, or go to the bathroom! Remember there are already over 3500 births a month in Jerusalem alone.

So, when the midwife/nurse wants to break her water and the mother turns to us with beseeching eyes saying, "Should I let her?" I want to crawl under that birthing bed never to come out. *"I told her not to ask me questions in front of the midwife."* It really does upset them. They went in to this profession to have a relationship with women not with the monitor. They also are the ones medically trained to make decisions. The doula is supposed to provide information to help the mom make a decision, but we aren't allowed to go against the medical personnel.

One issue here is that the midwives have rules to follow and policies to adhere to. In all fairness, they, unlike us, are the medically responsible personnel. So, doctors learn the technocratic model of medicine and we learn a natural, traditional midwifery model of birth. Today in Israel it is changing and it is refreshingly wonderful to attend a birth with a midwife whose horizons have been widened.

Most doulas, lay midwives and midwives from midwifery schools in Europe and America believe in the body as a whole unit. We don't separate the emotions and mind from the body. Some caregivers don't appreciate the beauty, power and sanctity of birth. It's a pity that they spend as much time with paperwork as they do with the birthing mom. It shouldn't be this way. When modern technology and high-speed computers are supposed to make our lives easier and simpler, it has simultaneously complicated and made our lives more anxious with the worries of viruses and back–up paperwork. It has also deleted much of the humanism in our work. A caregiver used to walk in the room, talk to the client and ask how she was doing. Then it graduated to, "Hi how are you?" to the client while handling the monitor strip. Now, with monitor screens at the nurse's station, they scarcely walk into the room!

It is no wonder that when a mom-to-be brings a doula, there are twinges of jealousy, especially when she turns to the doula not only for support, but for advice.

So, when the following letter came out from the Midwifery Association after two more doula trainings opened in Israel, it was no surprise.

The Midwifery Organization of Israel has set itself the goal of strengthening the professional status of midwives in Israel. Midwives act by force of the Law of the Ordinance for Midwives in Israel, and [the organization] is a leading body in terms of professional independence. We, as midwives and as members of the organization, wish to promote the profession by encouraging the broadening of the midwife's authority and the development of her skills.

Lately we have been seeing unprofessional forces entering the realm of midwifery, due to the claim that the midwives do not have enough time to provide the birthing woman with overall treatment, and that therefore outside help is needed, such as a doula. As a result of that, there have been many requests from all kinds of colleges, asking that we allow "clinical training" of doulas in the birthing rooms. In regard to this, and based on the circular of the Director General of the Ministry of Health (No. 14/03, from 18/3/03, 20 Av 5763), it must be remembered that a personal attendant of a birthing woman is not permitted to give treatment. The Midwives' Organization supports clinical training only of professional teams from the nursing/medical realms, and sees overall supportive treatment as being an inseparable part of the profession of midwifery.

The technological development and the complexities of treatment present midwives with new professional challenges, along with the increasing demand for one-on-one treatment and a personal approach. The solution, therefore, lies not in bringing in outside, unprofessional personnel, but rather making sure that the number of midwives in the birthing rooms will be in keeping with the number of birthing women. In addition, the Midwives' Organization makes sure to update [its members] constantly, and encourages the development of programs to broaden the skills of the midwives, in order to respond to these demands.

In light of all of the above, the Israel Midwifery Organization re-emphasizes the responsibility and authority of the midwife to provide physical, mental and emotional treatment for the birthing woman and her family. We therefore call upon you, the head nurses in the hospitals, the section head nurses, nurse in charge of birthing rooms and all midwives, to allow only people from the realms of nursing/medicine to enter the birthing rooms as participants in learning programs and clinical training.

Help us to preserve and strengthen the professional standing of the midwives in the State of Israel, who are legally licensed, and who carry the responsibility of global treatment for the birthing woman and her family.

Wow! I was speechless. Who could have caused such a letter to be distributed?

Unfortunately, the hospital-based midwives do not carry out global treatment. They aren't allowed to. They are not allowed to be hired privately as the doctors are. Some are so fantastic, women want to hire specific midwives for their births but the system doesn't allow it.

When I ask why not, I am told there would be inter-staff jealousy. Then I wonder why the doctors are allowed. Some are hired constantly over others. Isn't there inter-staff jealousy there too?

I'd never gotten answers to my questions. I only knew that when the doulas work peacefully with the midwives without stepping on their toes, the atmosphere was wonderful, the births exhilarating. Most doulas tried to keep the atmosphere friendly. I was sure this letter and other complications would eventually blow over. I shared this with doulas in the hope that we would remain stable and cohesively work with the staff. I would not take off my rose-colored glasses.

Chapter 21
Doula-ing Spills Over into Mothering

"I'M NOT TIRED!" one son declared.

"Can we finish the game?" shouted two siblings from their bedroom.

"Can I have my shower later?" another child asked.

I tried to be a bit flexible about bed times. "Your cousins come so rarely. Of course you can stay up later." Or, "That book has you really captivated. You can finish this chapter," I said, giving a kiss on the forehead.

The hardest time to wind them down is the first week after changing the clocks to summer time.

Sometimes there is fighting when they are cranky. *Little House on the Prairie* is not always our scenario, despite how I long for it.

I had to think of an idea to make the transition easier.

Walking off to my bedroom, I reached in my birth bag, pulling out the relaxation CD's and lavender oil. Going back to the kitchen, I opened an upper cupboard where I kept different sized candles for various occasions. I pulled out a lavender-scented candle I had bought at the Dead Sea on our getaway. I lit it, adding two drops of my lavender oil to the candle, hoping it would fill the room with even more fragrance.

Dimming the fluorescent overhead lights in the living

room, I carried the lit candle to the dining room table. This room actually doubled as our living room with a couch along the back and a rocking chair on the side. I walked over to the CD player, pressed the button to pop it open, and inserted the CD.

"What's going on Mom?" my ten year-old asked.

"Hey! What's that?" asked my five year old as he came closer to the table.

"This is what I do when I am at a birth," I answered. "It helps calm down the lady who is having a baby."

"Let's try it out," I said. "A couple of you can sit on the couch. Another can sit on the rocking chair. Someone can take a couch pillow and lay on the floor."

My three-year old giggled, grabbing a pillow from the couch. The rest scrambled for a place to sit. I continued, "Take a deep breath through the nose and release through the mouth. Watch me. It goes like this." I closed my eyes and breathed deeply hoping they would follow. I saw one follow, but the rest were either skeptical, too young, or thought I was plain crazy. I begged them to try, telling them it usually works.

After three minutes, not wanting to push my luck, I counted backward from five. "Five, four, three, two, one. Okay, you can open your eyes now."

One said, "That was cool Mom." One giggled. The others didn't comment.

Now, almost every night, like brushing their teeth, the routine was candle, music, story time and sometimes—it's too expensive to do daily—aromatherapy. The evening atmosphere was certainly calmer.

Once my daughter asked, "Can you give me a massage? I know you do that for your ladies."

"Sure thing, sweetie," I answered. "Would you like the ladybug or the roller massager?"

The evenings when I was off to a birth, Moshe sometimes took over. He told the bedtime story.

I bought extra CD's for our home so I was not stuck without them when I ran off to a birth, forgetting to return them to my birth bag. Tears filled my eyes when I thought of how supportive my family had been.

And now…the ultimate test. My own daughter, Nehama, was expecting my first grandchild. My twenty-one-year-old, brown-eyed beauty was growing into motherhood before my eyes. This quiet, calm, go-with-the-flow second child in a family of six was becoming a mother.

I was so proud of her knowledge, so grateful that she was aware of much more than what her grandmother knew, or what even I knew. My daughter knew, for example, that the gender of the baby is determined by the man. She would not have to feel guilty, like my mother did, when she had three girls. My mother lived with the feeling that she had disappointed my dad by not birthing the son he always wanted. My daughter was not ignorant of the childbirth process, but rather she became an informed participant. She attended an eighteen-hour childbirth series, which included readings and videos that supported the normalcy of birth. I sent her to an educator whom I knew prepared women for making informed decisions. I hoped that my daughter, prepared with the relevant information, would not passively lie through her birth, or receive an unnecessary episiotomy as I did, simply because it was hospital "protocol".

Nehama, which means comfort, is an Orthodox Jew. She believes in G-d and knows that whatever the outcome, she trusts that through Divine Providence, whatever will happen, will be for the good. She made efforts to have the safest outcome like eating well and exercising but ultimately, we are not in control. I was so proud and yet so scared. So proud because she is who she is and she wanted to do what was right. So proud that my stomach aches when she borrows another birth book to get more information and increase faith in her body. Tears filled my eyes when she asked, "What are my options? Should I have a homebirth or a hospital birth?" I gave her information, statistics and stories. Pros and cons, internet web site addresses and an informative book about homebirth helped her decide.

Her husband, who is a very supportive man, said, "I am nervous about a homebirth and feel safer in a hospital." He felt more comfortable with the machines that go "ping", setting off an alarm if a woman changes position. He was less nervous knowing there would be doctors around. Frustrated, I gave in to the wishes of her husband.

Nehama said she felt safe with me by her side, wherever she was.

My son-in-law respected my knowledge and his wife's desires, but she was still unsure. She also wanted to do what made him comfortable. He decided to consult with his rabbi.

A rabbi, in the world of an Orthodox Jew, is there to guide people in making important decisions with long-range consequences. For example, educational issues are often discussed with a competent rabbinic scholar who knows the family and their needs well. So, when it comes to an essential decision like where to give birth, I was not surprised that my young couple wished to consult their rabbi, who happened to live abroad. They would soon be traveling for the Jewish New Year, and hoped to ask him in person. I was nervous, wondering whether or not he had access to enough evidence-based research about the birthing "scene" here in Israel, and whether he had been apprised of recent studies showing the safety of homebirth. I wished I could be there myself, armed with all the relevant facts!!

A week before they left, I had a conversation, in my head, with my son-in-law about things that I didn't feel comfortable telling him directly. "I don't want my Nehama to lie there with a monitor for twenty minutes so the insurance company will be satisfied if there is a lawsuit. OK, she is now allowed to stand with those tight belts if the read-out strip is fine. What if they are too busy to come back to attend to her? Then what? Another twenty minutes? Do you really want her to get intravenous fluids that she doesn't need?" There was no response in this imaginary conversation, of course.

On one hand, I was so thrilled that our Jerusalem hospitals boast over 3500 births a month, but on the other hand, the busy staff can't always provide what the mom wants or needs. If she chooses to have her baby in a hospital setting, I'll pray that we are given the right person to help her attain her ideal experience. Even with this ideal person she won't be able to get what I long for her to have. I want her to have individual one-on-one care with a highly skilled midwife. I want her to have a quiet, calm, and listening ear. I want her to have total flexibility of positions. Unless there are complications, I want her to have intermittent monitoring with no interventions like breaking her water. I want her to have her baby in a secure, almost germ-free familiar environment. I suppose I want her to have a home birth; the home birth I never had; a birth where she feels really in control and in touch with her body.

She and her husband flew to Europe to be with his family for the holidays. They returned in good spirits, along with the rabbi's decision. "You can have a homebirth for subsequent births but not for this one," was his advice. "An untried uterus," he cautioned.

That's usually the term given by medical personnel. I was quiet, trying to disguise my disappointment, but Nehama felt it anyway. "It's okay Mom. You'll be with me." My heart sunk. I know loads of hospital staff. Most doulas get along well at the four major hospitals in Jerusalem, but there are still many midwives who feel we are on "their turf." We would be at the mercy of their medical decisions, unless my daughter felt she could make her own demands. Usually birthing women aren't in any condition to disagree with the authorities. This isn't something I want for my daughter!

I couldn't fall asleep easily that night, as I struggled to come up with an alternative plan that would be acceptable to everyone. A couple of weeks after they returned, I had an idea. I knew a midwife practicing at a hospital who would possibly do something unconventional. The next morning, after making a few calls, I reached Leah. "I know there are no in-hospital private midwives, but I want you to attend my daughter's birth."

"When is she due?"

"Another five weeks. The pregnancy is going fine, thank G-d. She is healthy and feels positive." Leah requested Nehama's paperwork and asked that my daughter call when she was in labor. Nehama registered in the hospital where Leah worked, which was not my hospital of first choice.

One month later, a week before her estimated due date, Nehama called me. "I have been feeling contractions all day but nothing serious." My daughter's voice sounded relaxed and content. She always had a high threshold for pain. "I just want to give you a heads up, in case this is real labor".

"Oh, I am so excited, "I responded.

"How are you feeling, sweetie?" I was starting to feel protective.

A couple of hours went by and I couldn't resist calling her to ask how she was doing.

"Fine, Mom. Mostly lying on the couch."

"Do you want me to call a midwife, Abigail, who lives near you to come and check your dilation?"

"Okay. That's good."

"It is a bit early to call *your* midwife, Leah, who lives far away."

I called and was happy to hear that Abigail was

available. She agreed to check Nehama. "Wait till my kids are in bed and I will come over. Tell her about 8 o'clock."

What a blessing. Abigail has such a warm and comforting presence, I was always so grateful to see her on shift whenever I arrived at the particular hospital where she worked.

It was so helpful to have someone who lives in my daughter's area that agreed to check the laboring women in their home.

"Do you know how many people take the forty-five minute trip into the city, many with a taxi, only to find they aren't in active labor? They walk around the hospital for two hours, are checked again, only to discover they are finally three centimeters. They are sent home and told to return when the contractions are every four to five minutes." This was what I told Abigail when I insisted on paying for her help. "You are really providing an important service by agreeing to check someone at home, and save them that big trip if they aren't that far along. Later that night, Abigail was on the line giving me the report: "Nehama is doing great: She is 100% effaced and four centimeters."

"Wonderful. Can I talk to her?"

Nehama gets on the phone, "Would you like me to come?" I asked.

"It's okay Mom. You don't need to come."

Wow! She was really chilled out! I decided to speak to Abigail privately, while she was heading home. "She is coping quite well, but I see it is getting difficult." She advised me to head out soon, since it was almost an hour drive to the hospital from her house and 45 minutes for me to get to her house. I would make the trip to my daughter's before it became too difficult. It was already 8:10 p.m.

Before I left, I called our midwife, Leah. There was no answer so I left a message.

Then I called my daughter. "Nehama, I would like to start over to your place. I can hang out in another room if you want."

"Okay, Mom." She agreed. "That's fine with us."

On the drive to her community, Leah returned my call, "I worked all day and I have day shift tomorrow. I just can't do it," she apologized.

I was stunned. "But we only registered in your hospital because you would be there," I tried to protest. "I don't feel comfortable with all the staff there!" "Don't worry. I will call to find out who is on shift."

Pulling up to Nehama's home, Leah called back to tell me who was on night shift. She told me the names of three women, two I barely knew and the other I was not fond of.

"They are both coming on shift from 11:00."

I was not impressed. Oh no, now what? She tried to convince me that one midwife was really very good, but I was still uneasy.

"Thanks," I told her.

"Good luck."

Now what do I do? My daughter was depending on me.

Knocking lightly, I entered to see her lying on the couch with the lights dimmed. She said, "The contractions are starting to hurt."

Around 10:30 p.m, I suggested that we wait until the shift changed at 11:00 p.m. We were ready to go. As my son-in-law drove, I updated Nehama that Leah wasn't available.

"Whatever you decide, Mom."

Ah! I hate when a client says that except this time it was my daughter! She didn't want the bureaucratic hassle of changing to a different hospital, so we forged on with the original plan. Personally, I was ticked off and went forward, with trepidation, as I tried to hide my true feelings. This was one of those times when I wished I had insisted on changing hospitals.

Arriving with Nehama at six centimeters, we were led to the delivery room, like any other patient. To my further consternation, I didn't recognize the midwife. Or the doctor! Nehama reached eight centimeters quickly.

While her labor was progressing quickly, the pain in her eyes was saying, "Help me Mom, this is too hard." I couldn't take seeing the desperate look. Shocking myself, I heard myself asking for the anesthesiologist. *Me? I couldn't believe it. So what if she is having a hard time? She didn't want to use medical pain relief and I certainly didn't want her to risk it! What were these words flying out of my mouth?*

But now she wanted an epidural. Actually, she didn't want an epidural. She wanted it not to hurt so much and just end already. They had broken her water sometime after we were moved into the delivery room. I didn't know when or why. Nehama remembered someone saying she was "stuck" meaning labor was stalled. *How could that be? I thought. We had been in the hospital less than three hours!*

Then, suddenly, there were decelerations of the baby's heart on the monitor. The doctor wanted Pitocin to progress the labor and was readying a vacuum for delivery. She even threatened a cesarean. Standing next to the midwife while she was attending to the delivery, the tension in the room was immense as decisions were being made about my daughter and my first grandchild. The monitor showed more decelerations, but the baby was coming quickly.

The midwife said, "Push hard, Nehama!" as she reached for the scissors.

"I am getting the vacuum ready," the doctor insisted.

I darted a pleading look at the midwife, glancing at the vacuum.

The midwife called out, "But the head is almost here!"

Nehama was fully dilated. My head turned towards the doctor, then the midwife, then to my daughter then back to the midwife. While I felt handcuffed, I wanted to hit the scissors out of the midwife's hands! "Don't you dare!" I wanted to scream. But my vocal cords were as anesthetized as my daughter's torso. I wanted to protect her and I couldn't. I was here as a mother, not a doula, but I could be back in this hospital as a doula next week and this could be our midwife or doctor. They would remember me as the interfering doula or maybe just the hysterical mother.

The midwife, with a glance at the doctor, then back at me said. "I am sorry but I have to do this."

I was fuming. The baby was almost out. There was nothing I could do.

A moment later, at 3:30 a.m, my first grandchild, a healthy baby boy was born, screaming and pink. Now I was needed to help my daughter's transition into motherhood. I would have to deal with my emotional state later. I could console myself by thinking *at least the vacuum and cesarean were avoided.*

I decided then and there that I was not cut out to attend my daughters' births. It was too emotional an experience. I was not "in charge," as Nehama thought I would be.

A few months later, my other married daughter, Nehama's older sister, was due to give birth. This time, I would make sure to hire another midwife who works as a doula, so I could come as just the mom, with some massaging thrown in. I knew my daughter, Tsippy, had a much lower threshold for pain, taking Advil (ibuprofen) to cope with terrible menstrual cramps since the age of fourteen. I knew she wasn't opposed to having an epidural though in theory, she wanted to hold out for as long as possible. I knew she wasn't my "ideal" client.

At Tsippy's birth, we were together most of the day until Joyce, a midwife, came to help her through the birth process. I had a gut feeling that I would need help on the home front well before we would leave for the hospital. She massaged, monitored the baby, and checked her dilation. Unable to cope with the pain, we headed for the hospital.

"If I am more advanced, I won't take an epidural. If not, I want one. Mom, I can't take it anymore," she said with tears flowing down her face. Arriving at the hospital when she was three and a half centimeters, with close, painful contractions, she received pain relief less than an hour later. Her face seemed a mixture of relief and guilt as she longingly looked at me for validation of her need for pain medication. "I'm sorry Mom. I just couldn't anymore," she said.

"Tsippy, it's okay. You're tried. You took it and it is working well. Now relax. I love you, sweetie."

She was fortunate to jump to ten centimeters in two hours. After twenty minutes of pushing, she delivered my seven and a half pound granddaughter over an intact perineum. Whether I liked it or not, my daughters were accepting of their births. It was *I* who had to work on my feelings. And I wanted to almost swear "never again." Maybe other doula mothers can handle going with their daughters as the doula, but I, for one, cannot.

Chapter 22
The Bathtub Birth

AFTER ACCOMPANYING ETTI to six out of seven births, our relationship was more than client/professional. We had become friends. I had attended her celebrations after her babies were born, met her extended family and attended births of her siblings.

Etti's labors followed the same pattern. She labored at home for a few hours before calling me. I joined her in her home and a short time later we proceeded to her private doctor at the hospital.

While attempting to handle the one-minute long contractions, which came every two minutes during the last hour of her otherwise easy labor, she attempted to answer the questions asked upon arrival.

The intake was handled by the nurses. "How old are you? When was your last period? Do you or your husband smoke?" There were about twenty questions altogether, the answers to most of them were in the file she had brought with her.

Etti detested that part of her labor. She was trying to focus, trying to cope. However, this was policy. The information must be documented.

We spoke last time about changing hospitals and doctors but she said, once again, "But I really like Dr. Rubin." My heart sank. We were now on birth number eight and she still wasn't aware that she could make different birth choices. Spreading the word is only as good as a woman's decision-making abilities. We had discussed her options but changing the familiarity of a particular doctor and hospital is unnerving for many women. They also may not realize how much better the experience can be.

So, one Monday morning when the phone rang at 7:00 and I heard Etti's voice, with a bit of sadness. I thought, *"What a pleasure being with her despite the mire she is stuck in."* Arriving at her house, I found her in the bath. I dropped lavender and orange aromatherapy oil to surround her with the fragrances she enjoyed. After placing the cassette into the recorder, my hands started the "double-hip squeeze", the only physical help that kept her from asking for drugs. I leaned over her as my hands found the spots on either side of the meatiest part of her hips, I pressed inwards. My knees were slightly bent to relieve pressure on my back. Her husband was busy scurrying the children off to school and arranging the babysitter for the eighteen-month old.

While with Etti, we continued our slow-paced breathing together during contractions while catching up on news in-between. This was still the early phase of labor. When she was at a more advanced stage of labor she preferred quiet. As I refilled her drinking bottle, she removed herself from the bath to relieve herself.

By 9:30, Ari, at Etti's request, called Dr. Rubin letting him know that they would be heading to the hospital in a few hours. "No problem", he responded, "I am already here working in the department."

As Etti's contractions finally were close enough to really consider leaving for the hospital, she asked, "Can we wait a bit longer?" They were four minutes apart but there was no traffic now and the hospital was fifteen minutes away. I never see a reason to arrive too early; however Etti's face showed signs of intensity which weren't there earlier. I reminded her how quickly the last hour goes, jumping from five centimeters dilation to ten. "Yes," she responded, "but I hate the hospital; the intake, the commotion, them telling me what to do."

I remained quiet, finding it difficult to disagree with her pleas.

"Okay, let's wait a few more minutes," was all I could say.

Ten minutes later, she quietly murmured, "What would happen if the baby suddenly descended and I have to push? Is there anything you need to deliver the baby?"

Ah-ha. *Now I got it. Subconsciously or not, Etti wanted to birth this baby at home.* "Etti, I am not a medical person. I have no equipment with me—nothing! Even if I did, this is not within my scope of practice. I am a doula, not a midwife."

Inside I was in turmoil. How could I allow this to unfold before my eyes? My heart whispered, "Let her have the birth she deserves!"

My brain said, *"I am not a qualified home birth midwife. What could I do if there are any complications that a midwife is trained to handle? We have to go now!"*

"Ari, please call an ambulance," I said.

Ari, from outside the cramped bathroom calmly said, "Okay."

Etti answered, "Not yet! It isn't time."

The conflict raged within me. She obviously wanted to stay home.

"Etti, please call a homebirth midwife. It may not be too late."

I knew good and well that there were none who lived in the city. The closest one lived a twenty-minute drive away. But maybe there was a midwife in the city. One never knows.

"Great idea," I heard from outside the bathroom door. "Can you give me a couple of numbers?"

While I passed Ari numbers, praying someone was in the city, Etti stated in a quiet but certain way, "My waters are opening. I am sure they broke."

"Ari, you have to call an ambulance!"

"No", said Etti."

This is the stage where Etti began to tense and by now, usually in the hospital, her doctor asked her to get on the bed in the standard position.

I had tears of joys in my eyes as I watched her, in a standing position, knees a bit bent, as she bore down taking charge of her body and birthing the way she wanted. I had to admit I was proud of her. I pushed away the fear that we were being irresponsible. There was no time for self-chastisement.

"Jane is on the way. She was interviewing a client in the city", exclaimed Ari. "She said she doesn't want to come because she doesn't have her birth kit with her."

I shouted back, "Tell her I have no supplies and I am

a doula. She has nothing, but she is a midwife!"

"She wanted to know if there are any medical issues," Ari continued to shout.

"None," is all I answered; there was too much going on right now. I kept this conversation short and sweet.

Right or not, Etti was not moving and they weren't calling an ambulance. I breathed a sigh of relief knowing Jane was coming, even though I was well aware that there were only minutes before this baby would be born and she may not make it. "Etti, blow for a few minutes to give Jane a chance to get here." She quietly shook her head "no." I saw I didn't even have time to put on gloves. (After taking two courses to learn how to handle an emergency delivery, I was told to carry a pair "just in case"). After two pushes, a pink, baby boy slipped into my waiting hands. Etti was in a state of euphoria.

"I don't believe I am standing in my bathtub holding my new child," she exclaimed with joy. I gently placed Etti's son into her arms, keeping the baby at the level of the placenta. Ari passed me a warm towel from the dryer, a precaution I had learned. Rubbing his little back to dry him off and to make sure he continued a good cry, I didn't truly relax until I saw Jane walk through the bathroom door.

Jane arrived in time to attend to the cord. "I am so glad you could come." After helping Etti wash off, which was easy to do in the bath tub, we guided her to her bed, keeping her newborn wrapped in warm towels. Etti breastfed her son while Jane attended to the placenta. Ari brought Jane a container to save the placenta in. The eighteen-year old babysitter returned with the eighteen month old, putting on a happily surprised face when she heard the good news and saw the new baby.

Jane made sure the uterus was contracting normally. Then she stepped outside the bedroom to give the parents their time for bonding. I gave Jane an embrace with a big "thank-you" for running to meet us. Smiling back she replied, "I am all for choice but can you just plan it a bit earlier next time?"

Chapter 23
Spreading the Word

MY EARLIEST MEMORY of myself was the friendly little kid who said hello to everyone. I wasn't shy. There was Rose, the crossing guard lady near my elementary school. She was rotund with pink cheeks winter and summer. From when I entered kindergarten, I warmed up to her right away, giving her a daily hug. To a five year-old, she seemed ancient. On one of my trips to visit my mom in Philadelphia, I went to the grocery store, passing my old elementary school. Tears came to my eyes when, thirty years later, there was Rose. "I bet you don't remember who I am," I said to her.

She answered, "I do because you were the one who always smiled and said "hello" day after day, year after year." She remembered my hugs too. "I am retiring this year," she added. After thirty-five years, it was enough. She must have been thirty when she began. So much for "ancient." We hugged and wishing her luck, we departed.

So, strangers attracted me, especially when I was spreading the word about doulas. I would talk about our profession anywhere and anytime. When I read in DONA's magazine that May was "International Doula Month," I just smiled. For me, every day is "International Doula Day."

How many times I have entered a taxi on the way to a birth, when I started a conversation with the driver? "To such-and-such address," I would say in a hurried voice. "I am on my way to a birth. I am a doula. Do you know what that is?" "I think I heard of that. What *exactly* is that?"

Entering into my emotional rather than statistical explanation on what a doula is about, I explain how long we have been around, and how we assist a couple with their positive birth experience. Our ride speeds by quickly. When the ride is long enough, the driver, whether thirty or sixty years old, shares the stories of the birth of his children.

One conversation went like this: "You are coming home from where?" the forty-something taxi driver asked.

"I am coming from a birth. I am a doula, labor coach. Have you heard of that?" I asked.

"I think I read about it in some newspaper once. What exactly do you do?"

I went into my usual explanation about our emotional and physical support to assist a woman through labor.

"We also provide information and help the couple to advocate for what they desire written in their ideal birth plan." I added.

"Wish I had had one of you when we were expecting our third." He said. "My wife went for a test that the doctor highly recommended she take because she was thirty-five years old. She did this test that checks the water around the baby," he continued.

"Amniocentesis?" I asked.

"That's the one."

"Well, we were told everything was alright and that we were having a boy after two girls. That night her stomach wasn't feeling right she told me. Bleeding began and by the next night she wasn't pregnant anymore. We found out later that the test she took can have this possibility, even though it is slight. Maybe they told me but I don't remember if they did."

"I am so sorry." I said.

Once, when a computer technician came to fix a technical problem, part of my code had the word, doula in it. "You know, "labor support" I said to him. This is the term also used in Israel. Then I said "doula" in a heavily accented Hebrew. Some have heard of it when pronounced this way.

"You have children?" I asked.

"Yes, one, five months old".

"So, how was the birth?" I asked.

"Traumatic, I almost fainted near the end."

Thrilled I was not paying him by the hour; I asked if he wanted to explain. The next ten minutes we spent on my favorite topic, birth.

"My wife gave birth before she even took a course. At thirty-four weeks, she went into labor. It was long and hard. I did what I could until she took an epidural. Then I got to cut the cord."

Wow, I thought sarcastically. *What fun!* "My wife went into a depression the night she came home, three days later. No one talked with her, supported her or helped her. We were always an independent couple and they thought we were managing. Her mom lived in another city. She could only take off from her job a month later. I was stressed taking care of the shopping, cooking and cleaning while trying to cut down on working to help her."

"How long did her depression last?" I asked.

"Two months. I am told we were lucky. My brother's wife was traumatized from her first birth which ended in a cesarean. She now has only elective cesareans. She is pregnant with her third. She didn't even want to try a vaginal delivery after the first birth. My brother was down about it but happy that she still wants more kids."

He didn't know the details of the birth, but he understood enough to tell me they could have used assistance. "A doula," I said. "No promises, but a doula could have helped."

How many times do we hear about women who chose a cesarean over a vaginal birth? Part of it is for convenience. The mom wants a certain doctor on a specific date. Also, induced labors cause women to opt for pain medication much too early in labor, throwing the whole system out-of-sync, leading to cesareans, especially for first time moms (primips). When forceps are used and a nice size episiotomy is cut, there is little chance of a woman to attempt a vaginal birth the next time. The birth was too traumatic. Coupled with the fact that many doctors and hospitals do not want to give a trial-of-labor (time-intensive and exhausting with unknown time of delivery), a cesarean is scheduled, making it easier on everyone involved the second time around. Yes, easier on everyone *except* the mother. There are complications that surgery entails, infection, increased blood loss, respiratory complications, risk of additional surgeries, and more. Complications for the baby are also well researched. It is normal for a child to be born through the birth canal.

"Do you know that when a doula attends a birth," I explained waiting for the PTA meeting to begin, "there is a lower chance of a cesarean?" While waiting in line at the bank, pizza store or even at my daughter's graduation somehow, when I am around, the word "doula" enters the conversation.

Chapter 24
Life Cycles

"THERE'S NO PLACE like home." Well, Dorothy, you were right. But, my mom's needs outgrew her home. Her rented, two-bedroom apartment, one block from my house, had been ideal. She could be looked after by Beth, her new live-in caregiver and I could pop in any time to check on her. Was she eating well? Feeling cold? Stiff? Needed a massage on her legs, stiffened with less movement? I could easily get the answers to any questions I wanted to ask. Unfortunately, when the phone rang at 5:00 a.m. one Rosh Hashanah morning, I wasn't so sure it was the "ideal" situation. Seeing my mom's number on the caller ID, I flew to her house, just about changing out of my pajamas. She was choking and coughing. "I wanted to call an ambulance," said a shaking Beth. After ten minutes, Beth and I calmed her down, gave her a drink and avoided a trip to the hospital.

These crises, most of them less dramatic, sometimes put stress on my nerves, resulting in stress in my home. I needed my husband to pick up the slack when I was busy with mom, at a birth or to help with mom's paperwork. The sun set way before the work is done. The book called *"The 36-Hour Day"* was a very appropriate name of a guide for people taking care of relatives with Alzheimer's.

Mom's apartment with narrow doorways, too narrow

for her newly-acquired wheel chair, was impossible to navigate. Since it was a rented place, I had to ask the landlords about breaking doorways. "No," was their reply. "Don't touch the apartment even if you return it to the way it was."

My mom's need for space and her occasional screams in the middle of the night which disturbed the neighbors caused us to seriously think about moving her into a nursing home. She would soon need two caregivers, one for night and one for the day. She would need someone for Sundays when they were both off. We could see that round-the-clock help was on the horizon. I began to search for an old-age home. We would have to make the move before her contract expired in two months.

Between Mom's situation and the following story, I began to philosophize about life and also about death.

Last week I attended Judy's birth. The labor of her fifth child was difficult, birthing a son who was quite large for my petite friend. He was eight pounds five ounces with the labor and decent was not less-than-volcanic movement. The midwife was stupendous as she encouraged the birthing mom onto her hands and knees, while manipulating the large baby's body out of the birth canal. It was a skill- a true work of art. On a cold day in late November, as the winter solstice comes closer, I witnessed a spring day. Judy's birth was the catalyst that pulled me away from slowing down, from rejuvenating at a time when it was needed.

Then, one week later, the phone call came.

Judy's dad had a massive heart attack. He was buried yesterday and now she was sitting Shiva. Shiva is a seven-day period when life stops. The mourner does nothing: no cooking, no cleaning, no driving, no personal care. It is not only a time to slow down; but a time when life comes to a complete halt. Judy, who had just brought forth life, now had to think about death. Her dad knew she had a baby, and then he left this world. When I visited Judy, she had a chance to share feelings about her dad behind the tired eyes: tired eyes from birth or from death? Emotions wreaking havoc on the system: the elation of a birth, the sadness of a passing, a journey into this world and a journey into the next. Judy simultaneously bore witness to life followed by death. At rare times like this, I become philosophical.

As life renews itself like a seed, there has to be a breakdown before the growth. As nature slips into the seeming "decline" of the year's cycle, when fall becomes winter, with leafless trees and rains or snowflakes begin to fill up the lakes, I am surrounded by renewal-birth. Doulas anticipate the next birth or at least *I* do. When two weeks go by and the phone does not ring, my body begins to yearn for the adrenaline rush, as well as the frantic pace of putting a quick dinner together, throwing a load of laundry in the machine, and a big hug to the children, and spouse, if he has managed to get home in time. Maybe this isn't for all doulas but it certainly defines my life.

Life cycles are supposed to ebb and flow. This is the nature of the seasons, the nature of life itself. So, I looked at my calendar to confirm the estimated due date of my next client. In the meantime, I had other responsibilities and privileges to attend to, including my mom.

Chapter 25
Dancing with Mom

I WENT TO visit Mom one rainy afternoon when she wouldn't be able to enjoy her balcony. She loved the view overlooking the forest. This was one of those days when a visitor would really be appreciated. Maybe a Scrabble game would be nice, even if I have to throw the game so she can win. Actually, it was hard even to do that anymore. She knew she'd been making no-brainer words with few points so we didn't bother to keep score. Compiling two or three letter words kept her mind challenged and at least she was playing her beloved scrabble! Three months ago, the last time we played, there were more misspelled words than not.

I knocked on the door, letting myself in. "Hi, Mom!"

"Hello!" she answered. Her speech was becoming more minimal with the progression of the disease.

Sentences got shorter. Nouns became "that thing" and "this thing."

I gave her a kiss and told Beth that she could take off for an hour.

Placing a Mel Torme CD into the player, I asked "Do you want to dance?"

"Sure."

Mom always loved to dance. That was how she met my dad-at a USO dance for soldiers.

When I was thirteen, and my mom was forty-one, she registered for a tap-dance class. Ginger Rogers always made it look so easy. She kept her old shoes in a shoe box in the basement dreaming of her favorite movie stars and how she danced a bit like them. The shoe box became her hiding place for bank bonds which Alice, my sister, found after packing up my mom's belongings. My mom forgot she'd hid them there.

So now, Mel Torme was singing on the CD and, taking her hands, I said, "Let's dance."

Mom smiled as I began, "One, two, three and one, two, three." Moving my feet as if I remembered how to polka, Mom shuffled her feet trying to follow. The blind leading the blind. I began to smile and we both began giggling.

"Forget Mel Torme!" I said. Then I started singing the song from the *King and I*. It was one of our favorites. "Shall we dance, one, two, three and..." We started to "dance" the polka, not knowing who was Anna and who the King. I held her hands and watched her smile as she enjoyed the movements. "One, two, three, and."

Suddenly Mom stopped. Her head tilted to the right, then to the left as her eyes focused on my face. Her gapped-tooth smile widened with curiosity as she said, "Who are you?"

Stunned and speechless, my eyes filled with tears. The answer did not come right away. I knew it would happen one day. I read it in the books. The literature prepares the family of Alzheimer's patients. They write information like "No throw rugs, they can trip" or "bars for stability when bathing."

But no book can prepare a daughter for this. I knew one day she would not remember me but I thought that day was far in the future. The future had just become the present.

"Mom, it's me. Sarah," I choked the words out.

She continued to smile, but her presence seemed absent, staring as if I were a stranger. I decided I would dance-we would go on. I could keep dancing with my mom! She is enjoying it so much and, for the moment, that is all that mattered.

Chapter 26
Spreading the Word BIG Time

AS THE CHILDREN began to grow, getting busier with their own lives, I seemed to get vacuumed deeper into the world of birth. There certainly was a lot of cleaning up to do; generations of women lying on their backs to push out a baby, routine interventions, and cesarean rates had skyrocketed to over 33 percent.

A few years ago, I began receiving calls from a few miles away, asking if I have such and such a book. "Yes, I do," was my answer. "But I live in the northern end of Jerusalem."

"Oh." A quiet pause on the other end of the line.

"I will try to get it to you."

"Thanks."

Sometimes the women were on bed rest while others worked full time. Most had no cars. Logistically, my home was not an easy-access location.

I decided to open libraries! I asked my rabbi if I could use ten percent of the payment I received from births I attended for the purpose of purchasing a wide selection of informative books for the pregnant woman. Usually this tithing goes to a cause - the poor, blind, widowed, orphaned. He agreed that disseminating information was an important cause which could help the public.

"Hi," I said to an old client, totally surprising her. "I

want to open a birth library in your community, but I need someone to house and operate it. Interested?"

"What is involved?" was the question I always received.

"It will give women an access to a plethora of the most recent pregnancy and birth information without them having to spend a lot of money!"

Some friends and ex-clients were inspired to help "The Cause."

After opening my first two libraries within the year, housing 10 books each, I occasionally received a call asking, "Do you have a book with birth stories? I don't want a book on pregnancy and birth, just stories."

There were no birth-story books available for the observant Jewish woman. We needed something to read for emotional and spiritual strengthening.

"No, I am sorry," was my answer each time.

Then it struck me! I certainly went to enough births and was told enough stories to write my own book. I had never written professionally because I had nothing to write about. After I was asked about a birth-stories book, I was inspired!

I picked up the phone to a publishing house in Jerusalem to find out what was needed.

"I need some money to help fund the book," I told Moshe. "They aren't willing to take a chance on an unknown author."

"I don't know if we can afford this. See what you can do by brainstorming with a couple of birth buddies," he encouraged me.

After calling a close friend not involved

professionally in birth, she agreed to help me with the project for a low wage.

That would keep my budget low and give her some income.

Malka and I got together to write a fundraising letter. It was addressed to old clients and some colleagues as well. Malka came over a couple of hours a day to organize the mailings and some phone calls while I opened up the computer to start typing birth stories.

Leafing through pages of notebooks, where I documented births, I wracked my brain to remember details.

"Hi there, Susie! I am writing a book of birth stories and yours was so inspiring. I wanted to write in a couple of details that you may remember."

"I am so honored. What do you want to know?"

"First let me ask you if you want it to be anonymous."

"I think it is fine to put our names in it, but I will ask Yonatan when he comes home later."

"Okay, then let's talk about the birth."

Other times I scrapped a particular birth. Not enthralling enough. Then I put out the word that I was looking for other birth stories. I wanted ones from generations ago and even other countries. E-mails came in and some snail mail letters too. I continued attending births. Arriving home at 2:00 a.m., I would then write.. The story was fresh. I was too keyed up to go to sleep anyway. For more than two years, all I was thinking about were birth stories. During those two years, I opened, with support of others, three more birth libraries in areas around Jerusalem. In 2004, my first book on birth, *Special Delivery,* was born. There were stories from two generations ago, from different countries, a taxi birth and a birth after years of infertility. It was a book of information, entertainment and inspiration.

The feedback on my book kept me motivated to collect more stories for a future book, which was to come out three years later in 2007. There was a lot more medical information as well as the usual inspiration. The calls regarding the libraries urged me on to open more in other communities. I also expanded to the Hebrew-speaking market with books from Janet Balaskas and Sheila Kitzinger which had been translated years before.

Chapter 27
Scissor-happy

ONE MORNING AT 7:00 a.m., I received a call from another doula, Esther. She was attending a birth when she got a call from another client. "Can you take over a phone call? The woman is hysterical and the labor barely started! She may need me before I finish."

"No problem. Give me her name and phone number and I will assess the situation."

"I just have to warn you: She has hired Dr. C." Esther knew my feeling about Dr. C. He was the head of the department and a very skilled doctor. Unfortunately, he was also a very busy one. I had yet to hear of a primip (first-time Mom) who hired him who did not receive an episiotomy and/or a vacuum. When I attended births with women who had him previously, this was what I was told. When doulas met at conferences to share information regarding caregivers for our clients, Dr. C.'s pattern was discussed frequently. "Who should Mimi hire?" I would ask someone. "She wants the head of the department at such-and-such a hospital."

Another experienced doula responded, "If she doesn't mind an episiotomy, she can use him."

We really try to keep a "Code of Ethics" in our work, but we must inform our clients so they can make an informed choice.

Racing through my mind were the recent studies I read. Trials regarding episiotomy vs. tearing were drastically different. For first and second degree tearing, there was quicker recovery, less pain, and less damage to the sphincter muscles.

I was not excited about attending births with Dr. C., but now there was no time to waste.

"Hello, Mina. This is Sarah G. I am Esther's back-up."

"I can't talk," she said as she gasped for air, passing the phone to her husband.

"Hi. This is Shimmy. Her contractions are coming every two minutes and are long, strong, and extremely painful. She is throwing up and has diarrhea."

"These are definitely signs of a precipitous labor. You should head for the hospital. Hope I make it in time."

As I drove to the hospital, I got stuck in morning traffic. Crawling along worrying, wondering if I *would* make it on time, I reviewed my past encounters with Dr. C.

Following the technocratic-medical model of care, Dr. C. was very typical in his approach to birthing women. I remembered our last conversation.

"Why don't these women take epidurals?" he asked me.

"They don't want to have medication in their bodies when they give birth. Also, there is a high risk of slowing down the labor when taken too early." I added.

"That's okay. We can add Pitocin to speed up the labor."

"Then if the fetus goes into distress?" I asked.

"No problem. I will do a vacuum." he assured me.

"Don't you have a protocol at this hospital that all primips who have a vacuum have to have an episiotomy? I asked.

"That's right but then we sew her up. She is as good as new," he answered with a grin.

"Hmmm. Well, most of my clients prefer to avoid interventions, if they can be avoided."

Traffic. Too much traffic. There was no driving in-and-out of the bumper-to-bumper traffic. I took a different road. Signaling left, I was off on the old road that no one used anymore. Great. I was moving along at a fast clip. Suddenly I reached a fork which joined up with traffic coming from outside the city. Crawling along, I prayed to G-d to get me there on time. Popping some relaxation music into the cassette, I took some deep breaths to calm myself.

The usual twenty-minute ride took forty minutes.

I reached the reception room and asked the midwife, "Where is Mina Gold?"

"She is in Room #6," she answered pleasantly.

Hurrying to room #6, I knocked and entered. Mina was lying in bed with her legs in the foot rests and her newborn on her stomach. Dr. C. was about to cut the cord. Dr. C. said hello with his usual Mona Lisa smile.

At 7:50 a.m. he clamped the cord, gave instructions to the midwife to deliver the placenta and turned to leave the room.

"Wow! That was fast. Mazal Tov, Mina!"

"I can't believe I gave birth so fast," she answered.

"How long were you pushing?" I asked.

"Only once! The baby flew out."

I glanced at the midwife, who I'd known for years. She saw me glancing at the used scissors on the tray by the bed and understood my questioning eyes, which asked, "Why did he cut?"

She pantomimed to me so the new mom would not understand, picked up the oil bottle, used for perineum massage, and signed, "I tried to give him some almond oil but he shrugged his shoulder and picked up the scissors."

I could not say another word to Mina, an innocent victim of an unnecessary procedure.

Walking to the door of the room, my back to the birthing mom, I fought to hold back the tears.

Following me to the door the midwife whispered, "If they hire him, they should know who they are hiring. The baby was five-and-a-half pounds and an episiotomy."

I didn't know this young couple. It was the first time we'd met. If she'd been my client, I would have explained to her the options and the facts I know about her doctor's delivery style- episiotomy and sometimes vacuums. I would have suggested she call for more references. Maybe Esther did and Mina chose him anyway.

I took a deep breath, forced a smile and re-entered the room.

Glancing at the clock, I saw it was 8:00 a.m., time for the daily doctor's meeting. Dr. C. was the head of the department, so he had to be there, hence the episiotomy to speed things up.

"I wish he would come already to stitch me so I can put my legs down," Mina complained.

"I'll go ask the midwife to tell him," I responded, trying to hide my sadness.

Ten more minutes passed and he was still at the meeting.

Mina was very sore and uncomfortable, her open cut still bleeding. Doctors do the stitching here in Israel, especially if they are hired privately.

I left the room to find the head midwife. "Where is her doctor?" She is lying there waiting to be stitched," I said firmly. "This is his *private* patient."

Ten minutes later, Dr. C. entered the room with a smile on his face, flanked by two residents. He proudly proclaimed in a voice that sent shivers up and down my spine, "I cut an episiotomy because it is so straight, so clean. Makes stitching so much easier."

The residents; one man and one woman, looked at him passively. As he raised his hands in the air, he said "Like a tailor creating a hand-sewn suit," pulling the imaginary needle and long thread upward. "If we don't cut, she could tear apart like an explosion," he said, removing his hand long enough to motion sideways to emphasize the danger.

Taking a few minutes to stitch he followed with, "Look at how nice it looks. As good as new."

The residents stare with fascination as he finished his sewing job. I wondered if they realized her flesh will never be like "new."

"But Dr. C., when I go to the birthing mom's home for a postpartum visit, the women with the episiotomy have a lot of pain and trouble sitting. The women who have a tear seem to be walking more easily. They hardly complain of pain," I boldly ventured to comment.

"Could be," was all Dr. C. says.

Shrugging his shoulder and patting her thigh with a "Mazal Tov," Dr. C. exited the room.

Chapter 28
Hope Springs Eternal in a Doula's Heart

A WOMAN HAS four hospitals birth options in Jerusalem. Each one has a different ambience. At 5:00 a.m., one Sabbath morning, I received a phone call from a client who had chosen a hospital that is not so "doula-friendly." The interaction there had deteriorated in recent years for three reasons: the staff wanted a closeness to the birthing mom without a third party, doulas had spoken up in lieu of the couple (a no-no), and doulas seemingly got paid much more for the *short* amount of time she is with the couple. They don't realize how much time we put in before and after the birth. Many don't know how many hours we are supporting them at home before we get to the hospital.

This particular Sabbath, my married daughters, with their children- my four adorable grandchildren - came to visit. I had been looking forward to their twenty-five hour visit, because we lead such busy lives and they live out of town. I don't get to see them as much as I wanted to. My preparation began Wednesday, preparing traditional Sabbath delicacies: kugels; potato and vegetable, four vegetable salads, a chicken in wine and spices, fried schnitzel and of course, the traditional Sabbath chullent, a stew with all types of vegetables, barley and meat thrown in. It simmers overnight on a hot plate and is served for lunch.

So, when the call came, a prearranged taxi driver drove me to my client's home. My client called for him to pick me up, so I did not have to make the phone call on the Sabbath.

I put a warm smile on my face and ignored my pangs of disappointment as I left my family behind.

I arrived at Ruth's home. Her water had broken three hours earlier. The contractions were coming four minutes apart.

Great! Maybe I would be home for lunch!

Helping her through the next couple of hours of labor, she was not ready to go. The baby's head had been low all week, the water was clear and there were fetal movements. The contractions came closer together.

I opted out when Shmuel, Ruth's husband said, "How about some chullent?' I'm not hungry. I was not eating chullent at 8:00 a.m., especially while thinking of my family back home. After Shmuel ate, they decided to leave.

Arriving at the hospital of her choice, she was told, "You are barely in labor; about two centimeters open and the cervix is 70% effaced."

We were having an interesting day as I tried not to think about my family back home waking up, going to synagogue to pray, eating lunch, going to the park with my grandkids, and hanging around. Once I was with Ruth and Shmuel, I had to be with them mentally, too.

After a monitor and questions of all sorts to record, we went to a birthing room. As Ruth got into a shower, I hung around while Shmuel passed out in a reclining leather chair. Two centimeters. I didn't believe it. I wanted to go home.

Hearing sobs, not from a birthing mom, I noticed a doctor, who I will call Dr. Yael. Her cries and yelling were coming fast and furious from the direction of the nurse's station. I heard her say something about bringing a substitute and how she can't take it. "I have been here ten years and I am tired of this!" she cried. It sounded as if she was an over-tired, stressed-out doctor. Her medium length brown hair, slightly covering her face could not hide the worn, tired face and watery eyes. She went into the staff kitchen which had an entrance with no door, next to the delivery rooms, exposed to all.

As I was refilling my client's hot water bottle at the urn, a midwife growled, "If you need something, ask us. Otherwise, stay in the room."

Later, my parched throat led me to venture out for some tea, and the hot water bottle turned cold. I peeped out to see if anyone was available. There was no midwife in sight. So, walking to where the hot urn was kept, I saw Dr. Yael in the staff kitchen. She had gained her composure by now, but what choice did she have? We had worked together in the past. She seemed to be here every time I came. Asking her permission to enter the staff area, she said "Sure."

"I couldn't help but notice your strain. I wanted to give you a hug, but it didn't seem appropriate. As woman to woman, I just wanted to say I am sorry for your pain."

"Thanks."

She seemed open to my staying there so I continued.

"I read a book called *From Doctor to Healer*. Heard of it?"

Shaking her head she asked, "What's it about?"

"It speaks about different models of medical care: technocratic, humanistic and holistic."

I continued to explain the transformation of the doctor's journeys.

It was so nice to talk to a doctor as a colleague, sharing information that can make a difference in our common cause to help women birth better. She asked if I could find the book for her as her English is very good. Tomorrow I would make it my business to order a book for her.

The day wore on; the sun was setting as I had long given up on seeing my family. Ruth was having a difficult time as she took seven hours to go from two to four centimeters, well after her water had broken.

She asked for an epidural and I was asked to leave while it was administered. I left right away as Ruth was really in a lot of pain. The contractions had been every three minutes for many hours. She gave it her best.

By 9:30 p.m., when stuck at ten centimeters with the baby's head at -2 station, I asked the midwife, the third we had since arriving, if we could please have ten minutes without the monitor. Nothing I tried until now seemed to be working. They didn't allow much movement so I couldn't try anything too radical. Anything I would try would make the monitor reading inaccurate. "I want to just try something I learned from a Mexican midwife named Naoli. She described positions to help a labor progress if the baby was stuck. It should only need ten minutes."

Removing the monitor, she watched as I folded the hospital sheet in half lengthwise and half again. I didn't have a Rebozo, the colorful Mexican scarf used for this attempted "procedure". Improvisation is a doula's job.

Having Ruth go onto her hands and knees, I placed the sheet underneath, pulling it through on the other side. Raising up her stomach while forcefully pulling it to one side, we paused only for a contraction. I was trying to lift the fetus out of the pelvis so it would engage into a better position. There were no guarantees, but we needed to try. We all wanted to avoid the operating room. We continued for ten minutes.

"Pressure, I feel pressure," Ruth cried out. The midwife came in to check her. To everyone's joy, she announced that Ruth had advanced from -2 to +2 station (a term used to describe the descent into the pelvis) Excitement filled the room as the midwife opened up the birthing packet and two contractions later, caught a baby boy.

Dr. Yael needed to do some stitching, so she came into the room. Our glance was obvious only to each other that we shared a secret. I left with a positive feeling that the world *could* be changed, if only one birth at a time.

Despite some of the friction in this particular hospital, albeit not with every midwife, there had been a slow change after the harsh letter written from the Midwifery Association a year ago. Through e-mails and conferences, we had been able to liaison, attempting to make the atmosphere in the birthing room calmer. The whole incident and whatever caused it was beginning to blow over.

Chapter 29
The Second Getaway

AFTER MY SECOND book was finished and my mom was settled in her new "home," it was time for a celebration and some time off.

In the 2008 DONA International Vancouver conference, I heard topics entitled, *"Staying Fit to Doula"* by Stacey Scarborough and *"Mama Renew: Self-Care for Doulas and Mothers"* by Sarah Juliusson. They discussed a doula's 24/7 emotional and physical role which can be stressful. The main message was clear: take care of yourself or you'll burn out. Take time out physically by going to an exercise class or emotionally by going to a movie for a good laugh or a good cry. For a social rejuvenation, visit an old friend for lunch. Attend a lecture. So many helpful suggestions were offered. This advice was more appropriate for both a doula *and* a mother of many children or an adult child caring for an aging parent.

I had been under so much tension. "More insomnia, neck pains and stomach aches," I told a fellow doula. "There's an advertisement for a group trip to a hotel by the sea, three hours from our home," she shared. "Maybe they still have rooms available."

I had attended one of these trips a few years ago. It was invigorating!

Picking up the phone right after we hung up, I asked, "Is there any room available for the group booking next week?"

"Yes Ma'am, there is."

I was relieved to hear myself saying, "Please book two more for your three-night vacation." The receptionist asked the pertinent details and the deed was done! We would leave behind discussions about buying books and clothes for the upcoming school year, how to rearrange the bedrooms now that a teen would be in boarding school and my concerns for my mom who still had her wonderful caregiver, Beth. There was absolutely nothing happening that could not wait three days.

The three-hour trip was uneventful. I was so glad Moshe liked to drive. I slept and left him at the wheel. As we reached the shore line, about an hour away from our destination, I was roused from my sleep. "I am happy to see your calm face relaxed, no tension," he said. The lovely, expansive Mediterranean was a greenish-blue, with waves bouncing a boat which looked so tiny far out in the ocean.

"Want me to drive?" I asked.

"No, I am fine. Maybe we will take a break and walk a bit. My legs could use a stretch," he said.

Without speaking, we walked along the beach, inhaling the salty air and digesting the quiet.

I saw this was going to be glorious, three days of swimming, tanning, sleeping-in, and long, uninterrupted conversations with my life partner. No one would need me and if they did, it was great to know someone else would be good enough. While filling my body with good food that I didn't need to prepare or clean up, I would fill my soul with lecture tapes from rabbis who speak about how to achieve good character, how to tithe our money, and the beauty of the Sabbath day. This is a time for Moshe and me. It is *Just the Two of Us*, as the line from the old Karen Carpenter song says.

Chapter 30
A Different Type of Doula-ing

TWO YEARS AFTER Mom immigrated, she moved into a nursing care facility a 25-minute bus ride away. It went smoothly, being more traumatic for me than for her, it seemed. After two years of living in an apartment, a five minute walk from my home, I was sad when I walked past her old residence. I was not able to just pop in to say hello. Now, visits needed to be scheduled ahead of time. Sunday, when Beth, her soft-spoken Filippina aid of three years was off, was my visiting day.

It was also very sobering for me to realize that this was her last stop before death. Watching my mom deteriorate was very emotionally challenging. There were twenty-five people in the residence; each one dealing with disabilities caused by accidents, strokes, dementia and Parkinson's disease.

On a typical Sunday, I arrived at 8:00 a.m. to feed Mom breakfast, a simple act that she could no longer do herself. "Mom, you can swallow each spoonful of food slowly". Before giving her the next one I watched as she chewed. She wore a bib to catch the excess particles that dribbled down her chest. Our roles were reversed. I was nursing my mother who nursed me when I was helpless and vulnerable. "Patience"- a doula's #1 asset.

After breakfast, I pushed her in her wheelchair up

and down ramps, to enter the courtyard flanked with bushes bursting with red and yellow roses. I continued the walk around the home because the pleasant wind stroking her face relaxed her features. On rainy days, the hallways became our "treadmill" as a staff member and I supported her under each arm while she struggled to walk on her wobbly feet which used to power walk. We went back and forth with all our strength, supporting my 130 pound Mom.

"Physical strength" asset #2.

"Mom, doesn't this smell great!" I needed her to hear my voice that she never verbally answered. Sometimes the eyebrows rose and sometimes her head slowly turned towards me. "Intuition" - asset #3

The fragrance uplifted my thoughts as we sat in the garden together. We used to share this beauty together in the days when she could still focus. Now, she barely notices them. It brought back memories of the rose bushes my dad planted on Bergen Street over forty years ago. The deep red, bright yellow and vibrant pink bushes were a stunning forefront of our brick house.

Now, Mom and I sat on the balcony with the sun streaming on our backs as the shade of the trees partially protects us. I told her stories about her grandchildren, though she didn't respond to my words. "Little Miri and Adi are the sweetest little girls. Whoever would have thought I would have blond grandchildren?" "Instinct"- asset #4.

I held her hand, knowing that touch is crucial at this stage of her disease. When words meant little more than a soothing voice, touch was calming and provided her with the reassurance that she was still noticed, alive, and someone cared.

"Mom, Tova started a diet and Mendy is going to summer camp next week," I told her. I prolonged some chatter for her to continue hearing my voice. Loneliness was always difficult for her to bear. Now I finally understood why the TV went on first thing in the morning and she fell asleep to the radio. It was company for her, living alone for over thirty years. . "Empathy" - asset #5.

Feeding Mom a hot well-balanced lunch, I smiled and talked to her as I also stroked her cheeks. She returned a smile when I kissed her. When she ate the hot meal, I could see her chewing and swallowing with raised eyebrows and a smile. Her thin lips parted, as her teeth were exposed showing her three middle lower ones which had broken in half. She also bit her lower lip until it bled. The dentist said "Leave them alone. It's "normal" at this age." The staff said, "This is normal for Alzheimer's patients." I took her to a special dental clinic where they discovered her gums were infected and some teeth needed to be filled and others pulled. "Advocacy"- asset # 6.

There was another woman at the small, rectangular table where Mom sat. Her name was Esther. Esther had a stroke two years ago and had been in this facility ever since. She had difficulty swallowing so she ate only blended food. It was a consolation to me because Mom still chewed her food. Mom savored each bite. She didn't like the food that slid down easily. She enjoyed chewing. "Grateful" –asset #7.

Last Sunday morning at 6:00 a.m., I was called to a birth. But by 1:00 p.m., Leah had given birth, a quick uncomplicated event. I was happy to taxi over to Mom for the glimpse of what was left of our morning. I jumped out of the taxi running up the eight steps to the entrance of the home. A flashback of the movie *Tuesdays with Morrie* suddenly appeared in my mind. Years before Mom had become incapacitated, we watched the film together. It was a moving story about a relationship of a young man and his ex-professor who was suffering from Lou Gehrig's disease. The student, who had become a busy newspaper columnist never kept in touch with his professor as he'd promised. After seeing a news feature about him on television, he vowed, every Tuesday to visit him, until his dying day. The movie was full of philosophy and caring. My tissue box was almost empty by the movie's end.

I usually call our day "Sundays with Mom". After the birth last week, I bound breathless into her room. I found her lying in her bed, listening to Barbara Streisand singing "People, people who need people, are the luckiest people in the world." Moved to tears by the appropriateness of the words, I stroked her face to let her know I arrived. "Mom, I am here," I spoke to an unresponsive face, glazed eyes staring at the ceiling. From birth to this. "Adaptable" -asset #8.

I am grateful that Mom saved her money so that she could employ Beth. She helped take stress off me as well. With two professions; a mom of six children and a doula, having the security of knowing that when I dashed out to a birth, there was someone I could trust. There were also meals in the freezer. It helped me to sleep at night. "Spontaneous and organized" assets #9 & 10.

My family, when not in school and working, pitched in to help. My partner in life, Moshe, now had a flexible job so when I needed him he was there. When Mom needed to be taken to her special dentist or her wheelchair needed to be taken for repair, I could depend on him. He was also great with the documentation, banking and bureaucracy that overwhelmed me. My sixteen-year-old daughter, Tova, visited her grandma every week. "I really appreciate the massages you do for Grandma," I would tell her. "I am sure she does too!"

"Support network"—the largest asset and a must!

Chapter 31
Personal Life/Professional Challenges

I USUALLY LOOKED forward to this time. It is a time of introspection. It is a time to thank G-d for what we received during the past year and look at what we have accomplished. The New Year is a time to make resolutions. We try to apologize to people we think we may have wronged, and resolve to change and improve, especially in interpersonal relationships.

This year, however, I was more focused on birthing clients. I didn't want to disappoint them if I was at a family holiday meal or in synagogue, praying. My clients and I developed a relationship, albeit not as long-standing as families and friends, but an important one filled with emotion and dependence. They were counting on me!

I also did not want to sit down at the family meal with a married daughter visiting and suddenly, sometime after the soup course, say "Oh no. Sorry but my cell is ringing." They hear it too. We are all always hoping that we are not hearing right. Last Rosh Hashanah I had the same dilemma. The conflict was challenging: to be on call for clients or to be with my family. A doula doesn't have predictable hours.

All my children were coming home this year, including the son who lived at a boarding school. My married daughter and her husband were coming with my granddaughter. We were all dressed in new clothing for the holiday, my granddaughter in her pink flowery dress that I bought for her. With her golden, wavy hair flowing below her shoulders and her big blue eyes, she could be a perfect advertisement for anything.

My husband sanctified the day with blessings on wine as we stood around the dining room table watching the candles glow on the shelf in the corner. When my married daughters came, more candles were lit. Each of them lit one candle for each member of their family. My eight were glowing as were my daughters' three.

So, during the chicken soup course, as we were enjoying each other's company, my five-month-old granddaughter, falling asleep on my lap, my cell rang. "I haven't even cut into the matzah ball!" I exclaimed. Looking at my kids, and they at me, they said "Okay Mom. Hope you'll be back soon."

Another said, "We'll miss you."

Looking down at the sleeping beauty, I kissed her as I handed her over to her dad. As supportive as they are, it was difficult for us to say farewell since we had no idea when I would return. I had been trying to make great efforts to set my priorities at this time period. My obsession with birth for almost seven years had forced me to make serious decisions. I have had to choose between attending the wedding of a friend's child or a birth. Family gatherings were held a few times a year, usually at the holidays, so giving my clients black-out dates was not easy, especially since my back-up doulas do not want to take those dates either!

Other decisions also took place. Do I get six hours sleep so I am less crabby the next day or do I write at the computer to unwind when I arrive home at 1:00 a.m. after a birth? The passion and addiction to the high after attending a birth aroused a desire inside of me. I wanted to share with anyone who would read, through my writing. Needing to put pen to paper or rather, letters to a screen, I always wrote up my clients' births just for memory's sake, mine and theirs. The writing also allowed me to share my experiences with others when I published my work in various doula and women's magazines.

I started attending writing workshops before my first book was published and I pored over and dissected books about writing skills and techniques. At these writing workshops we were told, "To be a good writer one has to read a lot." My main reading material in my youth was action books, like Nancy Drew, the Hardy Boys and Alfred Hitchcock. I had to get tips, take more creative writing workshops, read the ten best sellers on the New York Times list and get a good editor.

My enthusiasm for birth extended into writing, which called for decisions which helped me balance my personal life and professional life. Now, wanting to publish these birth stories so other birthing moms could be inspired, I did a lot of late-night writing when the children were asleep.

The High Holiday is a three-week period of feasting, fasting and loads of guests. I was torn again because my book seemed to be so needed. Women asked me to expand my libraries to other communities. The libraries housed ten of the most updated books promoting safer births, exercise and nutritional information. I wanted to promote the knowledge that a healthier mother can birth a healthier baby.

Our family usually took a couple of day trips during this holiday season. Sometimes we headed north to see the mountains of the Golan Heights or west to visit my husband's aunt near the sea, but this year we were thinking of going south, either to the Negev or Eilat. It usually depended on the weather—north if it was hot, south if it was cool.

"I heard the weather forecast," Moshe told me one evening over dinner. "Cool weather is predicted."

"I suppose we are going south?" I responded

"Yes. The kids will really enjoy themselves. They have new tourist attractions. There are some antiquities with interesting coins and artifacts. There is also a new amusement park we can stop at on the ride back."

"Great. There will be something for all ages".

Assaulted by conflicting emotions, I tried to hide my feelings. I wanted to write! I finished reading a book by Natalie Goldberg, *"Writing Down the Bones."* She says "write, write, write." She continued, "Make a special place or don't make a special place; in a restaurant or forest, on a bus, or in a plane. Bring a tablet everywhere with a couple of pens."

Well, if I could go for my morning walk on the quiet black-tarred country road while reading her book, I supposed I could travel and write. The difference was that then I was alone, flanked by a mountainside on my right and a forest down the sloping hillside on my left.

This time I would be with family. My concentration level would be different as I tried to give my family some much deserved attention. Then my brain wandered; I was thinking of new ideas to write about. Pushed and pulled through setting priorities I could only tell myself that family time is crucial; it is what memories are made of, it is irreplaceable. *"Focus on the holidays and reconnect to spirituality."* I was feeling as if I had to convince myself of this. It can be any working woman's inner turmoil, setting priorities, professional and personal.

My professional passion must be put on the back burner to give to the people I love and who love me. Another few weeks would not matter in the scheme of life. Winter was coming. That would be a great time to hibernate in the warmth of my home and finish a book.

Chapter 32
Beyond the Call of Duty

SHIRA SAID, "I am sorry for waking you up when it isn't quite 6:00 a.m."

Putting on my glasses I saw it was 3:00 a.m. *True, it isn't quite 6:00,* I thought.

In our prenatal meeting, I handed them a paper with some information about when to call. I let them know that we are early birds and they can call as early as 6:00 a.m. so I can rearrange my day accordingly. "You may not need me until noon, but I like a heads up. My schedule works around yours." I explained to them.

"Hello Shira. What's up?" I asked.

"Well, I have been having contractions for a couple of hours and they are getting stronger. I think I am going to need you soon," she continued.

Good reason to wake me up now! I thought.

"Great! I will throw on some clothes. Should be in your house within half an hour."

Throwing on my purple lab jacket, I was on the way to the 10-minute walk to her house. I enjoyed the star-filled Jerusalem night, smiling as I thought of how convenient it was when a client lived nearby. I didn't need to call a taxi and the postpartum visit was easier to fit into my calendar.

The cell rang. It was Josh, her husband. Now I knew it was serious. "I think she is in transition," he said.

"I am right outside your building. Please call a taxi."

"But my mom will be babysitting the other two children. We have to wait for her," as his calm turned to panic.

"Where is she?" I asked.

"Two buildings over," he said.

"Don't worry. She will be here before the taxi. If not, our paths will cross on the way out." I assured him.

As we opened the door, his mother entered.

"Hello Grandma! Can you please bring me a large, dry towel from the bathroom?"

Handing it to me, we were out the door.

In the taxi, I spread the towel under Shira. It's a precaution I take to keep on good terms with the taxi drivers. It would be a big mess to clean up if the amniotic fluid opened up while he was transporting my client in labor and even more so if the baby came with it. It never happened in almost 1000 births I am happy to say. Four or five women gave birth in their home with an ambulance on the way, but never in a taxi.

"I feel a lot of pressure," Shira declared.

"Shira, when does your water usually break?" I asked.

"When the baby is ready to come."

"I am really feeling pressure," she exclaimed.

I told her to get on her hands and knees putting her head down in my lap. The less pressure on her bottom, the better.

"We won't make it to your hospital. I suggest we go

to hospital A, a five-minute drive. We just don't have the extra fifteen minutes." (We could change hospitals if we needed to.)

"I trust your judgment," Shira said. Her husband gave instructions to the driver to go to hospital A.

"I want to push," said Shira.

"Blow! Blow! Blow!" I calmly but firmly stated.

A big splash was all over me, the towel, and Shira's robe while passing the entrance to the hospital.

I called the hospital's delivery room. All four Jerusalem hospitals are programmed into my phone.

"We are taking her into the ER room," I told the woman on the phone from L&D.

Actually, the delivery was going to be in the taxi. She was pushing, an urge that is uncontrollable. I watched the head exit, the taxi pulled up to a halt outside the entrance to the ER. The driver jumped out searching for help. The husband was right behind him.

"Shira. I am putting your knee on the upper back of the driver's seat to be able to continue to birth your baby." I pulled down her long black robe trying to maintain a semblance of modesty. Thank G-d there was a bit of light coming from the street lamp outside.

At least I knew the staff was on their way, but the head was out and the color of the baby's face was turning darker. I whispered, "Everything is okay. You can push if you feel the urge." G-d only knows I have seen this almost 1,000 times. It was *very* different the first time I am doing it in the back of a taxi in the dark and in this awkward position. Her head was still on my lap while I am trying to reach over her bottom.

The shoulders were freed while I eased the baby onto the now red-stained white bath towel. The taxi driver was pacing and the husband, who had gone inside the hospital, was exiting with a midwife and some ER staff.

"It's born?" asked Tali the midwife.

"Yes it is. You want to cut the cord?" I answered.

We eased Shira onto the stretcher while the staff carried in her baby boy, who we found out later was 9 1/2 pounds, her biggest baby since her 8 1/2 pounder!

I wiped up the back seat as best I could, and wrapped the underwear in the towel.

"Someone is going to have to pay for this mess," said the driver looking at the back seat of his taxi.

"How much will cover it?" Josh asked as he took out his wallet.

"It's not just the clean-up, but the two hours of lost work."

"Whatever you want," said Josh as he handed him a few big bills."

Inside the hospital, I requested a plastic bag to dump everything, including her socks and robe, now that she was in a fresh hospital gown. After the staff finished the delivery of the placenta, I left to bring Shira a hot cup of tea.

We wound down by discussing the details of what happened and when and if anything should have been done differently. "I am very happy the birth went this way. I was at the hospital without the parts I don't like. It would have been nicer to get there five minutes earlier, but that's okay."

"I think ten minutes earlier would have been nice," said Josh.

"This was what was meant to be," Shira added. "This is the hospital I was meant to be staying in over the Rosh Hashanah holiday."

Picking up the bag of dirty laundry to hand it to Shira's husband, he looked at me and look down at the bag inquisitively. "Forget it," I said. "I will take this home and wash it out." Somehow, I could not imagine giving him this job, nor even his mom. This wasn't the first time I'd cleaned up after a birth.

Now he had another advantage of living nearby. He even got a laundry service!

As I loaded the machine at 5:00 a.m., I lovingly poured the soap in, knowing that this task was due to the birth of a new soul brought into this world. It was for something so special. When I hung the laundry later that day, I thought that this woman was not just a client. She was like my sister or a good friend. We had shared such an intimate moment. We birthed her baby together and for that, we would be forever bound. Hanging her laundry was part of that experience. Baking a cake for the circumcision ceremony would be another. Other doulas I know help prepare meals while others have older children babysit the siblings of the new baby while the new mom gets some much needed rest. Now "laundry duty" can be added to the list under job description for a doula!

Chapter 33
The Sandwich Generation

ONE MORNING, WITH everyone out of the house, I began to think about the kids.

I tried to include them in the excitement of the births. "Hey... flag a taxi!"

Arriving home I would describe the baby, "He was sooooooooo tiny," I'd say while holding my hands 12 inches apart. When I finished too close to dinner time, I called saying, "Pizza for dinner!"

With the joys of becoming middle-aged, I became the famous child in the "sandwich generation." That expression never had a negative connotation for me. Now I knew it meant more stress. It was a time when one married off children, sent others to college, helped with grandchildren and took care of elderly parents. Celebrations and responsibilities, albeit enjoyable and important, could be a challenge.

On top of this, add a job as a doula: work that is unpredictable, day and night, physically and emotionally challenging, and you have a recipe for a breakdown. It was uplifting to feel needed and wanted, but a mom has to try to find a balance.

Choosing the mode of transportation from the old age home back to my home was always a challenge too. Sometimes, I was so emotionally overwrought that the dam of tears threatened to burst open and I was embarrassed to ride on public transportation. In those times, I took a taxi home. If I drove there, then I wondered if it was safe to drive home with blurred vision and distracted thoughts. Usually, I took the bus there, so there was only the decision to make between the bus and a taxi. If the bus was my choice, then I hid in the last row praying no one I knew would sit next to me. I considered buying dark sunglasses for these visits.

On my way home, I remembered the debate some friends and I once had.

One, Esther, lost her mom in a car crash when someone hit them from the passenger's side, killing her instantly. Another friend, Susan, lost her dad after a debilitating seven-month illness.

I had a conversation with each of them, discussing a slow loss of a parent or an immediate one. Esther said, "It is so hard. I didn't say good–bye properly. I spoke to her every day. I just wasn't ready."

Susan said, "I am so glad I had time to say good-bye. Watching him die from cancer was horrible, but at least it was "only" seven months and he had morphine for the pain."

Then it was my turn.

"My mom's pain is horrible - the pain of losing one's mind, the boredom of not being able to participate in activities or conversations and the frustration of not being a useful human being."

Esther replied, "My mom would have hated that. She was so independent. Everyone needed her. She would not have wanted to burden others."

Susan just listened sympathetically.

I thought, *Mom can no longer hand out orange juice to people who donate blood for the Red Cross drives. Recording books to put onto tapes for the Library for the Blind is over. The television shows she loved are now incomprehensible.*

Then I added, "Her last bit of connection to humanity, the television and radio, were frustrating because they talked too fast, too loud, or too soft. Even her old favorite movies, now on DVD, were a cause of anger and confusion."

It was clear to me, from the expressions on Esther and Susan's faces that, like three judges deciding, the gavel was down- Alzheimers is the worst.

My mom could still enjoy handholding, kisses, and a hug. She turned towards us when we were nearby, noticed gentle voices, and occasionally recognized that someone was smiling. Oh, she didn't know who was smiling. It'd been a year since she recognized me, her daughter of fifty-three years. I had to be strong and go on.

I was so glad that Alice was coming soon. It made the situation easier to tolerate when someone was on the scene. Now I understood how alone she must have felt dealing with our mom. E-mail and phone calls were not the same as being there. Paula was not coming. We hardly have had any contact since I brought Mom here. At least she came for my daughter's wedding. The emotional pain with Mom being so far away was too difficult. I understood - I was in that same place. Also, she told me it was difficult being overridden regarding the decision to move Mom to Israel.

Popping into the old age home one day, as I passed it on my way home from a birth, I quietly walked into room #5. I watched her baby-soft face and her deep brown eyes which were closed after being fed her afternoon meal. As I sat next to her, stroking her face, she was relaxed. My eyes fill with tears as I watched. I screamed inside begging "G-d, let her talk to me!" I felt there was so much she wanted to say but couldn't.. Maybe her small stomach hurts because she was fed too much and can't say, "Stop, I can't eat anymore. I am a 125 pound lady."

Coming close to her, lying on her back in her wood-framed medical bed, I leaned close to give her one more kiss good-bye. As the babble passed over her lips, she moved her right hand conducting an orchestra that no one heard. I wondered how often she talks to herself instead of taking her siesta. Now I know why I found her sleeping while sitting in her wheelchair during the day. She probably hadn't slept much while in her bed.

"Mom, Mom," I called as her glazed-eyed face turned slowly towards my voice. "Mom, it's Sarah. I came to see you." Her slightly wrinkled face holding its age well, except for the jowls, turned towards my voice. Stopping midway into her 180-degree turn there was no verbal response. I straightened out the blue and yellow checked comforter, slipping my hands underneath to touch her feet, making sure they were warm. In the spring, the staff removes her socks but maybe they are cold, so I always checked. I wanted to be sure she was comfortable. In winter, I always made sure she slept with my cousin's hade-made purple and pink sleeping socks.

My cousin's mother, Aunt Mollie, is my mom's older sister. Eleven years my mom's senior, she, and her daughter are still taking care of my mom from 6,000 miles away, in whatever way they can.

Because she could not express herself, and tell us what her needs really were, caring for Mom was a guessing game. When she brought her hand towards her nose, I scratched or wiped it. When she moved back and forth uncomfortably in the seat of the wheelchair, I asked the staff to sit her on the toilet.

Now, lying in bed, her eyebrows rose up as I spoke to her. Her lips turned upward as I was yearning for her to say my name, which she hadn't said in more than a year. A tear flowed down my cheek, as I took her in my arms to caress and protect her as I do my newborn grandson; fully holding her in my embrace. Suddenly, in the midst of these loving feelings another dreadful thought arose. I had an overwhelming urge to take a pillow lying next to her and cover her face until there was no air left to breathe. Let me put her out of her suffering, and me, mine. I can't take it anymore!

No! No! I love her. I want her to live. I want her to get better. I want a miracle. The two conflicting thoughts waged war within me. "Mom! Look at me! Talk to me!" "Can you hear me? Do you know I am here?" Collapsing onto the chair beside her bed, I sat down and cried. I was angry at myself for those horrible thoughts, angry that my Mom had been reduced to a dehumanized pitiful subject. I wondered in agony, for the umpteenth time, *Why? This is a fate worse than death.* This was suffering for the patient and for the family. I know there is a rectification for every soul that is brought down and this must be hers but right now, I am not feeling so full of faith. My thoughts ran wild with despair as the tears flow down freely. I needed tissues. I got up to grab toilet paper from the bathroom that was mainly used only for showering. Who here needs a toilet? I returned and sat with Mom, holding her hand. I wanted to help her more. All I could do now was pray.

I finally noticed the clock on the wall reminding me that I had to leave. I had been here over twenty minutes. Had to go home. Had other responsibilities. Kissing Mom gently, I adjusted her head on the pillow. I backed out of her room staring at her new pink sweater-set fading into the distance. The color was so good on her. It added an illusion of life where there was barely any.

Chapter 34
The Induction That Wasn't

THE CALL CAME an hour before the Sabbath. It was my good friend from Safed, Briney.

"Sarah, what should I do?"

"What's going on? Why the phone call so close to the Sabbath?" I asked. I could hear the anxiety in Briney's voice. If anything, I was the one who would call her out of the blue wanting some parenting advice or to chat.

"My daughter, Rachel (living in Florida), is going to be induced by Monday if she doesn't have the baby by then. Her doctor won't let her go past the 41st week. Her other two births were induced so she took an epidural that she didn't really want to take and again there is another induction hanging over her head. She is really nervous."

"Not only that, her doctor won't take any responsibility for the baby if anything goes wrong if she chooses to wait."

"That sounds strange," I said. "Couldn't he just continue to monitor the situation daily?"

"It isn't so easy like it is in Israel," Briney said. "The doctor makes the decisions."

"OK. Calm down and we will think this through. Why is he inducing her exactly?"

"I don't know. That's what many doctors do in the

States. She gets an internal exam every week in the ninth month. She hates those checks. They are very uncomfortable," she continued.

"Why doesn't she refuse them?" I asked.

"She never thought about it. She goes to the doctor and that's what he does."

This was not the first time I have heard about it. This is not routine in Israel because there is no evidence to justify this procedure. If a woman has precipitous labors, gave birth in her car, or if she had a "silent labor" - *maybe*. A silent labor advances a woman's labor, without her feeling contractions. These are so rare I have seen this in three out of over 1000 births. It is certainly not justification for submitting women to this very uncomfortable exam, which can bring bacteria closer to the cervix or stimulate early labor.

I took a deep breath and said, "Get a pen and paper. Briney, I am not in favor and neither are the rabbis, of inductions unless there is a medical reason. I am going to give you a recipe for a natural induction, only because you are giving me no choice. I prefer to wait, if all indications show the baby is well, but taking castor oil is certainly safer than a medical induction."

"Thanks so much," said Briney.

"Here, we don't have as many reasons to induce as they have in the States. Either the baby is too big, the baby is too small, the water is too low, the date has gone too far, she is having twins, premature rupture of membranes, high blood pressure, maternal age and on and on. It seems there is little reason *not* to induce!" I continued, "This is not a matter to be taken lightly.

Inductions can lead to fetal distress, mal-positioned fetus, instrumental delivery, cesareans and more complications. There is also the spiritual aspect of a baby coming to this world when G-d deems it is time, not because of a 41-week gestation."

Ready to write, I gave her the recipe:

4 tablespoons (2 ounces of castor oil, 60 ml)

Mix it with a cup of orange juice

Stir well before drinking.

Drink one-third. After 20 minutes, another one-third. After 20 minutes, the final third.

"If nothing happens before Monday morning," I continued, "have her drink this mixture, and wait at home. G-d willing, something should start. If not, call me."

"Sounds gross," was Briney's reply.

"It doesn't taste bad, just a strange texture but it works almost all the time! And it certainly is much safer and less painful than a Pitocin induction. Good luck! Call me whenever you need to."

Monday morning, I got a call from Briney.

"Rachel told her doctor that she wanted to take castor oil," Briney began. "He said, 'Don't bother. It usually doesn't work and you will just get a stomachache.' She said she's going to try it anyway."

Tuesday morning. "Mazal Tov!" an excited voice bubbled on the other end of the phone.

"Briney, what happened?" I asked, mirroring her excitement.

"One hour after taking the castor oil concoction, Rachel ran to the bathroom with cramping and diarrhea.

Suddenly contractions began, strong and close. She told her husband to get her to the hospital, a half hour away. Twenty minutes into the drive he called a police escort who told them to wait on the side for an ambulance. Rachel screamed, 'Just get me to the hospital!' The police immediately called the hospital to expect her. They got there five minutes later. She sat in a wheelchair while her husband raced them to the elevator. As they entered, Rachel kept doing the "blow, blow, blow," to keep the baby in longer. The baby was born as the elevator doors opened. Rachel reached down and caught her."

"That's amazing. What a miracle! So glad I helped," I said.

"Thank you so much," Briney said.

The next day I called Rachel. "That was such a scary but wonderful experience. I hardly felt the baby coming out and the whole thing was over in two hours," she exclaimed.

"I have seen it take up to four hours for castor oil to work. Wow, you were quick! Were you fine with not having taken an epidural?"

"I never wanted to take one! I couldn't handle the contractions from the inductions! The only thing I would do differently next time is take the castor oil in the bathroom in the hospital and wait there."

Chapter 35
Making Inroads & Staff Relations Improve

A FEW MONTHS after our mutual birth and emotional bonding, I had left the promised book *From Doctor to Healer* at the nurse's station for Dr. Yael. I almost totally forgot I had ordered her the book until one day, out of the blue, my cell rang with a private number.

"Shalom. This is Dr. Yael R." I am sorry it took me so long to call about the book. I couldn't find your phone number."

"Shalom," I answer, surprised. "It's nice to hear from you."

"Thanks for thinking of me. I am sorry I did not respond sooner."

"Are you enjoying it?" I asked.

"English is not my first language so it is a bit hard for me."

"Take your time. It's yours to keep."

"Thanks again."

"Dr. Yael?" I began to ask a question.

"Yes?"

"I have one favor. When you are finished with it, please pass it on to other doctors who you think would enjoy it."

"I will do that," she answered.

I was so relieved that many years ago when the doulas were walking a tightrope, I and a colleague went to a famous rabbi to ask advice about how to handle this delicate situation. Doulas had been thrown out of a hospital because of "interference". His wise answer was "Go quietly and with refinement. You will get much further."

With belief in G-d and trust in my rabbis, I managed to handle many situations in life.

Midwives were becoming more accepting of doulas as we worked together often. As the natural midwifery courses were offered in different hospitals, I raised money to help fund one of them. When they held the course in 2006, they allowed me to speak on the topic of doulas and again at the 2009 course. Speaking at the previous course had motivated me to take the DVD "Doulas Making a Difference" and add Hebrew subtitles.

I also had translated DONA's *"Code of Ethics"* and *"Standard of Practice"* into Hebrew. Although most hospital staff, especially the doctors, know English, I had to make it user-friendly. They would certainly read it sooner if the papers were in their native tongue. Making a meeting with the head midwife at a hospital I frequent often, smile on my face and papers in hand, I said "Hello. I will make this short." With all the head midwife has on her shoulders, doulas were the least of her issues. "I have to keep my staff happy, the doctors calm and the patients safe." She had agreed to see me but barely remembered I was coming. It was no wonder. Her office, with its open door, was adjacent to the delivery rooms where there is always action and she is the supervisor.

"Come in, Sarah."

"Thanks for seeing me, Baila." (She prefers first name basis.) "The situation between staff and midwives has so much improved. I would like to see it continue. May I speak some time during this natural midwifery course about doulas?"

"Arrange it with Perla. She is the one in charge."

"Can I leave these papers with you?" I asked. "It explains what our code of ethics are and our standard of practice."

Her phone rang and someone knocked on the open door.

Taking the papers, we both stood up as I said, "Thank you."

"See you," she answered and she certainly would because my phone rang. It was a call from a lady giving birth in this very hospital.

I attended a second birth that began at 11:00 a.m. and finished at 11:00 p.m. The previous week's birth, a first-time mom, took twenty- three hours and I would appreciate a shorter birth this time. These are the labors that give us the stamina to keep going. I don't know any doula who could continue in this work if every birth were twenty-four, physically and emotionally spent hours. So, when Frieda, a second-time mom, called with contractions about five-minutes apart, we timed them together.

"They began only an hour ago?" I asked. "They seem to be a little short for now."

"Yes, but some are longer than others." she replied.

A bit later she called again. "Four minutes apart, forty-five seconds long," she declared.

I heard the deep breaths through each contraction.

I timed the next contraction.

Four-minutes apart, forty-five seconds long…Four minutes apart, fifty seconds long.

They were getting longer.

"Her husband, Baruch, is on his way home so you don't have to come yet."

"Why don't you get in the shower and we will speak in half an hour?" I asked. "Of course if the water breaks, the contractions get closer or you begin to feel pressure, call me right away."

Calling on schedule, Frieda said, "They are a bit longer and stronger."

Not wanting to take a chance with a usually quick second birth, I asked, "Can I come over?"

Without waiting for the answer, I knew would come, I grabbed my purple lab jacket and called a taxi. After arriving, I asked Baruch to put on the kettle. "A hot water bottle can really help for contractions," I said handing him the hot water bottle. I try to include the husbands whenever I can.

As Frieda placed her hand on her upper uterus, I asked her to describe the contractions.

"They are hard and they have been three minutes apart."

Going onto her hands and knees, she decided to do pelvic tilts while I pressed on her back with the hot water bottle, which Baruch filled to the perfect temperature.

Frieda's first birth was long and difficult. Her déjà vu

would not let her enter the hospital one minute before she felt ready.

When we went to the hospital, Frieda's heart sank as the midwife announced, "You are two-and-a-half centimeters with the cervix tilted back. Maybe you are 80% effaced. You aren't in labor."

The next few hours were spent walking steps, showering, and using loads of emotional support to help Frieda to forget what she had been through. This was a second birth, after all. It could suddenly pick up.

Two hours later she was three centimeters. Frieda was forty-two weeks pregnant, so she decided to let the midwife sweep her membranes to move labor along. "She is very disappointed," I whispered to the midwife when Frieda went out to tell her husband the news. "She really needs encouragement."

"I will be as positive as I can," said the midwife. And she was!

Four hours later she was a whopping three and a half centimeters. Tears trickling down her face, she said, "I just can't. This isn't for me."

Going to meet her husband outside, we begin discussing what to do next. Baruch reminded her that she didn't want an epidural. I reminded her that it is a bit too early to take it; cervix was still posterior and not fully effaced. "Let's try the shower again on the birth ball."

"Okay, I'll try anything."

The same midwife was still on shift. Bringing her a huge, blue physiotherapy ball, she said to Frieda, "This is the shleppy part, but it can pick up and move quickly."

What encouragement!

As Frieda relaxed in the shower, I asked her if she was ready for the baby. I saw she was so tense. "Let's try the relaxation exercises." As she breathed according to what she was taught in her Swiss Method, ante-natal classes, I gently touched her forehead, speaking to her affirmations for this birth.

We continued after she came out from the shower. Being a religious woman, she focused on G-d. "G-d is with you. His presence is at every birth. You are doing holy work. You are bringing a holy soul into this world to do G-d will."

Time to be monitored and checked again. "I can't! I just can't anymore!"

"I will only do intermittent monitoring," said the midwife. "The baby's heartbeat is reading out well so you can stay standing."

Six centimeters and off to the labor and delivery room. "I want an epidural. No I don't want an epidural. I don't know what I want!"

The midwife said, "You need to decide now or it will be too late." Ten minutes later she decided she wanted an IV to prepare for a "maybe" epidural.

Back to bringing G-d into the picture. "Let Him take over now. You are not in control. He can make it happen in the blink of an eye, just like the redemption, in the blink of an eye." We find the only CD in the player is one with religious Jewish music. "No fears now, you will finish soon."

Baruch was a great support.

As he fanned her, I pressed on her back, giving her sips of water while laying a cool washcloth over her face.

Baruch encouraged her, singing with the music and, between contractions, giving such encouraging words of support. "It is our baby that you carried all this time. I am so proud of you. You can do it."

Forty-five minutes later she was eight centimeters!

"I want an epidural," Frieda exclaimed. *A very normal thing to say in advanced labor*, I thought.

"You are almost there. Look how quickly you jumped!" I reminded her of *The Little Engine That Could*, a popular children's story that seemed very appropriate for labor. She liked it. "I think I can. I think I can," she repeated to herself.

The words were encouraging. Ten minutes later she was holding her little baby girl. She was ecstatic. "So glad it is over and that I didn't take an epidural."

The midwife said, "You were amazing!" Then she added, "Next time if you really want an epidural, tell us sooner so there is time to prepare."

Turning to the midwife I said, "I am sorry, but I tell them not to decide 100% *against* taking one or 100% *for* taking one. It is good to see how labor progresses and how they are managing, no?"

"I suppose so."

After the bonding and feeding time, I said good night, letting them know I would call soon. I entered the elevator on the ninth floor, pressing the button to the second floor to exit through the emergency rooms. At this hour, that's all that's open. As the lit numbers for each floor we were passing went black, the elevator stopped. Waiting a couple of minutes I realized I was going nowhere. Alone in the elevator, I pressed the emergency call button. A pleasant voice asked, "Are you alright?"

"The elevator isn't moving." I answered.

"I will send someone to help. Do you know which floor you are on?"

"I think the ninth. That's where I entered."

Waiting ten minutes, I pressed again. "Are you sending someone?'

"Yes, he should be there. Do you hear anyone outside the elevator?"

"No, not yet."

Thinking of my claustrophobic sister, I started to panic. *Well, it's me, not her,* I said to myself.

Then I decided to sit down. Crossing my legs in a tailor sit, I began breathing exercises. Sipping water and knowing I can talk with this strange woman through a speaker phone relaxed me.

Then I talk to G-d. *If You want me out of this situation, You will get me out.*

Think affirmations. Think positive thoughts.

At least I don't need the bathroom and I am not a lady in heavy labor who feels like pushing. I am in a huge hospital with staff that will help me out of here.

Fifteen more minutes passed, more quickly than I would have imagined. As security opened the elevator door, the guard said, "Sorry, but we had to check the electricity on the top floor before opening the doors."

"Okay. I am out."

Frieda's redemption. My redemption. Emotional panic attacks can be alleviated through support, techniques and faith.

Chapter 36
Mentoring

DURING THE NEXT two years, I wrote a second birth stories book for the Jewish woman. It had to incorporate what the first did not - loads of medical research of the safety of VBACs, homebirths, as well of the risks of inductions and cesareans. With two books now behind me, I decided to break out into the general population to help make the word doula a household word and to inform and empower all pregnant women. I was a locomotive train traveling on high speed to bring the passengers to an ultimate destination.

In 2004, I became a doula trainer and had taught eight groups. Okay, the first group had only three participants, but that was great for a trial class.

Now I had trainees who called for information and guidance. I held follow-up meetings so we could continue upgrading our skills and keep our connection.

Being a doula was great, but being a doula mentor was even more exciting. I could be involved with a birth without the loss of sleep. A doula would never call her mentor at three in the morning unless there is a real emergency.

It was also a pleasure to watch someone blossom.

"What does the teacher gain from his pupils?" asks

Maimonides. "The students increase the teacher's knowledge and broaden his heart."

Rachel, a mother of ten, finished my course. She lived three streets down the hill from me and constantly called with interesting questions. Now, mid-afternoon, she called to ask, "Can I borrow your birth ball later today?"

"No problem. I have no one in labor now. What's your lady's story?"

"This lady is having her fifth birth, but her births usually schlep for a while and then take off."

"Give me a heads-up when you are coming to get it," I told her hanging up the phone.

Calling me about four hours later, Rachel said, "I just called a taxi. The contractions are getting closer and harder. Can I come get the ball?"

"Sure. You pass my street on the way out. Where should I meet you?"

"Can you come to the bus stop? Oh, is the ball blown up already?"

Running to get the pump, I ran to the bus stop and was pumping away. Here I was with a huge blue ball and this pump. The pumps are hard to replace in Israel, so I didn't want her taking the pump with her.

I was so glad it was getting dark. I must admit I felt a bit silly doing this at the bus stop. As the taxi stopped next to me, the door swung open and Rachel gave me a big "Hello."

"Hi! Good luck!" The taxi driver had a curious look on his face.

I said quietly to Rachel, "Tell him about your profession and what this is for."

Waving good-bye, I motioned to her to call when it was over.

Another time I shared information with my class about a post-partum visit I had with a client. It was November when the weather in Israel cools off as we are heading towards winter. We don't have much of a fall here. There can be some pleasant weather with temperatures in the mid-seventies but it almost goes from the eighties in the summer, with occasional heat waves and cooler temperatures at night, to rainy and cold winters. The rain doesn't always come and we live with water shortages.

"When I went to visit B, her rented apartment with its stone walls was chilly," I told my class. "The windows are small, with the bedroom window very high up, at the top third of her ten-foot ceilings. The apartment is built on a hill and the owners had to improvise. The side entrance faces an alleyway which makes most of the house dark."

"My sister rents an apartment like that," a student piped up.

"Her two-year-old was out for the morning while her newborn was lying in her crib covered in a warm blanket. I glanced around after she welcomed me in. In these post-partum visits, I try to ascertain a few things - how the new family is managing physically and emotionally, if the nursing is going well, and if the baby's room is the right temperature. Most apartments do not have central air conditioning or heating so families have space heaters, electric or gas. B's apartment felt chilly."

"I can relate," said another student.

"We sat down to a warm cup of mint tea. Fifteen minutes were spent reviewing her positive birth experience. Soon after I asked how she heated the apartment."

"We don't have a heater yet," she answered. "We can't afford one."

"I gave her a present for the baby. She wanted to pay me my fee. Handing me an envelope with cash, I opened it and took 20% out of the envelope saying, "Use it for something you need."

When telling this story to the class, one student spoke up, "I have a heater we don't need. I will give it to her."

"That's wonderful," I answered. "I think she will have difficulty paying the electric bill. Can we take up a collection for her?"

After next week's class, we had a heater at her house with 500 shekels, enough to cover two months' electric bill. What a wonderful group of women.

This situation inspired me to buy a wall thermometer for my clients so they would know what the room temperature was. "Can you decorate it?" I asked my creative fourteen-year-old daughter who decorated it with blue and pink teddy bear stickers and white baby carriages, wrapping them in blue or pink ribbons. Bless her.

With trainees and new doulas like these, I could host meetings and workshops every few months with women who were inspired and enthusiastic. I didn't have to coordinate TALI (Doulas of Jerusalem) meetings anymore. If other women heard about a meeting and wanted to come hear the guest speaker, they could pay an outside, non-member charge and we would do all the work. It was a fair and a reasonable request.

When Selina, from my third training course, called to ask what she should do when her client was in what seemed like active labor, I asked for some history. "Well, I wasn't with her for her first birth, but after feeling some slight twinges, her water broke and she birthed in the hospital after half an hour."

"What's going on now?" I asked with trepidation.

"When I arrived, she was having contractions but no pressure. Then she told me the puddle by the elevator was her amniotic fluid, which broke after returning from the store."

"Yes, go on."

"I went to clean it up and returned to her apartment to find her with very few contractions that were far apart!"

I decided to let her work it out. "So, after comparing it to the first birth, what would you think she should do and what does the couple want to do?"

"She doesn't want to go," answered Selina, "but I think we should think about it."

"Did you ask if she tested for Strep B?" (This is a vaginal bacteria for which it is advised to take antibiotic in labor.).

"Oops."

"And do you know where the cord is or how low the head has been?"

"No. I have no idea," she answered sheepishly.

"Well, if she wants to stay home, it is her responsibility. I would encourage her to go the hospital to at least do a swab to see if it was her water and monitor the baby. They don't have to do an internal if she doesn't want one."

I feel a big part of my responsibility as a doula trainer is to be available to answer questions and offer guidance. It gives me a good feeling to help guide a new generation of doulas, passing on the tradition of women assisting women in birth. There is such a responsibility attached to giving out information when there is no one else to ask. Sometimes they call the childbirth educator when the doctor is not in the clinic. In the States, the couple calls the doctor's office and they say to come in. If they call the hospital because of broken water, they also would say to come in. Some private doctors here say the woman can wait at home if there are fetal movements and the water is clear.

"Come in when contractions get steady," one doctor told our mutual client.

Selina decided to clean up the "spill" while her couple packed everyone some food for the hospital.

Six hours later, three disappointed people left the hospital. They discovered that if her bag of waters broke, then it was a high leak, not a true break. One doctor said she was one centimeter and a nurse and another doctor said four-five centimeters during the five hours of being monitored and hanging around. That was a major difference! There were slight contractions. They advised breaking the water. "No. I don't want that."

Selina kept quiet. She wouldn't have minded getting

this birth behind her since she was already losing part of a night's sleep.

Picking up the phone to me, Selina asked "What should I do?"

"If she wants to go home, there is nothing you can do," was my answer. "Just make sure she has an ambulance number handy and you have sterile gloves to catch the baby," I said with a smile. "Goodnight."

One week later, I got a call. "Is a doula allowed to get mad? I mean, screaming mad?" asked Selina.

"Yes. Absolutely. It's a very emotional profession. What happened?" My empathetic voice stayed calm as my stomach started to rumble in anticipation.

"He just phoned. You know - the husband of my couple. She gave birth two days ago without me! I am so blooming angry!"

"Oh no. What happened? Did it go too quickly for them to call? Tell me what happened."

"Not really. I live a ten minute walk away," Selina continued.

"It was 2:30 in the morning when the contractions began. He didn't want to wake me up was what he said. They left some time later and she gave birth a half an hour after arriving to the hospital."

"So what do you make of it?" I asked, keenly aware of her disappointment and frustration.

"I just don't know. Maybe they decided the chemistry wasn't right or maybe they figured they could manage on their own. I worked them around my schedule this whole week, including taking a couple of afternoon naps, because I knew she could call any night!"

"Not only did I miss the birth, he asked if $100.00 was enough. I was taking $200.00 because I am newer in the field, but I was already with them for hours and lost a night's sleep. Now I missed the birth and we need to arbitrate over the payment."

"That always leaves a bad taste in the mouth. Did you have a contract?" I asked.

"I didn't have them sign anything because we live in the same neighborhood and I didn't think there would be a problem. I will go to my rabbi, who is also their rabbi, and whatever he decides, we will abide by."

"It is good to have a neutral person arbitrating. Let me know what happens."

The rabbi told the couple that they owed her the whole fee because they *chose* not to call her. It was not due to circumstances beyond their control.

Although there is a sample contract in the DONA manual, many of the doulas I know, DONA-certified and not, think that the contract makes this work seem more like a business than a calling. It has taken me years to be able to create a contract for a couple to sign.

Although it is a calling, I reminded myself and my students that it is a commitment from both sides. If all the conditions are written down, then there is less confusion, misunderstanding and hard feelings. Each side knows what is expected of them. If the client doesn't call or the doula sends a back-up, it is written clearly what will occur regarding obligations and payments. No surprises and no bad feelings.

The most exciting part about mentoring is when my student makes a suggestion that I hadn't thought of!

Our sages say, "I have learned much from my teachers and more from my peers, and from my students I have learned the most of all."

Making the Mentoring Worthwhile
Poem from one of my trainee groups

Dear Sarah
With a mixture of sadness and joy
With a feeling of achievement and pride
We come together for one last embrace
Before we hit the world outside.

We started out total strangers
Looking each other over at first
Each one so different from the other
But with a common desire and thirst.

To make a difference to someone
Somewhere at some time
To take a confusing situation
And give it reason and rhyme.

To give comfort and reassurance
To validate and connect
Replace fear and self-doubt
With courage and self-respect.

We are so different from each other
Yet we have all become friends

Sharing experiences, feelings and hopes
Planning together to make amends.

And who do we have to thank for all this
Who brought us together with a purpose and aim?
And gave us more than we ever expected
To her we rightfully give acclaim.

She went beyond the call of duty
With aromatherapy by Avraham Sand
Rina gave us a course on nursing
Nitza (PP depression group) taught-not everyone can withstand.

We were quite a rowdy group
Our yapping took us way off course
With questions and stories and personal accounts
We often took over the lesson by force.

But Sarah darling, patient and kind
Never lost her cool or got cross
Made each of us feel important
While securing her status as boss.

And so dear Sarah we present to you
A small token of appreciation
We hope it will match your doula get-up
And always give you a warming sensation.

Now don't think for a minute
That we have come to say good-bye

We'll call and badger with questions no end
For we trust that you will always reply.

Class of Winter 2008

I was very touched when my class presented me with a beautiful beaded purple necklace which perfectly matched my lab coat.

We would continue to rendezvous when I sent them notices regarding pregnancy and birth conferences taking place in Israel. Some of us reunited when *"The Farm's"* midwife, Ina May, came to share crucial information about the release of sphincter muscles for birthing. We also were informed about dream interpretation and how to use the Rebozo scarf for a non-progressive labor with Naoli, the Mexican midwife. I also organized learning sessions! We expanded our knowledge about aromatherapy, herbology, and physiotherapy for the pregnant woman. We also evaluated births that may not have gone according to "plan" so the students could develop their skills. The learning was fascinating and endless.

Chapter 37
Mothering the Mother

AS MY ATTEMPTS at "Mothering the Mother"—the title of a doula book that emphasizes the impact of a doula's work—became more frequent, my emotions heightened. We use this expression in our doula work as we "mother" the mother-to-be.

Visiting the old age home, I also "mothered my mother." When I visited, I saw changes in my behavior: "Hello!" I said to the staff. I started ignoring the posters and announcements of upcoming events while becoming more curious about the people. I didn't actually stare, because beyond their glazed eyes, maybe they knew I was looking. They were still with us, despite the fact we were not always sure.

It reminded me of when I scolded one of my children. "Did you have to leave the mess on the table?" The child being scolded turns away from me. Thinking, *"If I look away maybe my mom won't notice me?"* So maybe, if we look away, the residents won't be so needy, sad, and dependent on us. Maybe if we look another direction or sit and read, then we won't notice. But they *are* there and *they* do notice. They notice when, for instance, their nose runs and they need a tissue but there is no one to help them. Or worse, that there *are* people around and still no one helps.

One visit with my mom left me feeling raw and unnerved. It was Sunday, Beth's day off.

I arrived while a worker was showering my mom. Her high-pitched screams pierced my heart. Why is it so insufferable? These screams from the showerhead's spray on her skin were, for her "painful". Alzheimer's victims become sensitive to touch, sometimes not in a positive way. Or, we may know it is a shower but they feel like it is knives stabbing them. "Mom, please understand." And "Worker, make the spray softer."

The staff dressed my mom, a process that can take fifteen minutes and they just don't have fifteen minutes for each of the twenty-five residents. So, they showered quickly, with water running into her eyes and down her face. "It's only baby shampoo," they would tell me. "It doesn't matter."

"It *does* matter," I answered. "Just as when a two-year-old is showered, it's best to cover the eyes with a washcloth. Then it won't bother them. Then they won't scream." This was not the first time I mentioned this. It seems that some of the staff were better trained, others not, or maybe they were too rushed to get the next resident out for breakfast. The staff couldn't possibly tend to each individual resident with the devotion of a parent to a needy child. I tried to calm her down and to hold her shaking hand. I kissed her forehead and gave her a warm hug. Then I fed her breakfast.

After breakfast, I spoke with the head nurse. Between my birthing women and my mom, I was starting to feel like a professional advocate. "I know they were trained how to care for the residents needs but is there ever a refresher course?" I asked. I told her about the shower experience, explaining that when I have held a washcloth over her face, she did not scream. "I assure you I will supervise next week when Beth is off. I think she sometimes screams, even with Beth," she added. After a month of spot checks and me coming earlier, Mom's showers became much more relaxed, at least for now.

When Beth was off, my family took over. It was a very special but sometimes intense day because I was there eight hours straight. When I felt drained, I reminded myself *"This is my mom and there is only one. She fed me, now it is my turn to feed her."*

But the mothering was different this time. Mothering a woman in labor who was on the verge of birthing her child was the anticipation of a whole new family being born. Mothering a child who has his whole future ahead of him is a joyous time full of wonder and excitement. With a child, there is a sense of adventure as you hold your breath, anticipating his first fall while he takes those first steps. Helping my mom take her steps, I held my breath, and held on to her tightly, terrified that she may fall. Encouraging a woman to move in labor is a thrill as she works with her body to birth her baby.

As a child discovers the wonder of eating food, he licks his lips at the sweetness of the applesauce. Handing a laboring mom her food gives her the strength to endure labor. It is a pleasure to watch. Feeding my mom to maintain her survival aroused questions and doubts about end-of-life issues.

One of my daughters walked into the nursing home to visit and fed her ten-month-old son, while I fed Mom. I brought the teaspoon of pureed food to my mom's waiting lips while my grandson, Noah, almost jumped out of his stroller with anticipation of the food in front of him. My mom, sat staring blankly, opened her mouth only when the spoon touched her lower lip. Today there was no excitement, no joy. I only thanked G-d that she could still eat with a spoon and didn't yet need a tube or a feeding tube through her stomach.

I brought the spoon to her mouth. My daughter brought the spoon full of food to her son's mouth. She passively ate. He ate with eagerness. I wiped her mouth when the food spilled. My daughter wiped her son's chin as his food dribbled. Mom sipped from a cup. Noah also sipped from a cup.

Getting them to take their journeys took lots of encouragement. "You can do it Mom!" We helped her walk, holding her under her armpits as I, and a nurse, tried to get her to use her stiffening legs. "A bit more. You are almost there!"

Noah, with excitement and wobbly legs, tried to take his first steps. He had been holding onto the furniture as he attempted to walk around his home. "Yeah! Good for you. Keep going!" my daughter and I encouraged him. The only consolation when attending to my family is that my grandson is my future and my mom is my past. The birthing clients also represent the future.

As I wheeled Mom to her new room, my daughter wheeled Noah to his home, and the midwife wheeled the birthing mom to her room. The similarities were remarkable when I attended to all three of them. When Noah came to visit in my home, the flashbacks of feeding my mom came into my mind as I fed him. Noah in his highchair, my mom in her wheelchair and a birthing mom in hers, albeit temporarily. *Mothering the Mother.* A mother in a home or my grandchild in my home; different generations, different situations, but the same power of unconditional love.

Chapter 38
Car Crash at Midnight

AT MIDNIGHT, THE rings were inescapable. My cellphone, nestled in my feather pillow, pulled me awake. At this hour it meant only one thing — a birth.

"Hello, it's me," came the anxious voice on the other end. "Suri's husband."

Asleep only a short while, I was disoriented. "Who?" My head had hit the pillow only two hours ago.

"Suri's husband, Meir," he repeated. He continued to give me their address, a new one, and filled me in on the situation.

"I am throwing on clothes," I responded. "Should be there in fifteen minutes. Is everything packed?" I asked.

"We are ready. Just calling a babysitter," he sputtered out, wanting to hang up.

"I will call you when I am in the car. Thank G-d I have an earpiece for these situations so you can call me again if you need to."

I threw on my purple lab coat and headed to the car, feeling the drizzle of light rain, something we hadn't had for two weeks and sorely needed.

I warmed up the car before switching on headlights, defroster, and windshield wipers, I stared into the night. Two hours earlier, I was in bed, ready for a full night's sleep, and now I was trying to focus on the work at hand.

Driving down the highway at midnight was an eerie feeling. Sometimes I felt so alone, but at these times, I was thrilled. No traffic. Some lights blinked yellow at this hour, and the road was mine. I was glad I just winterized the car. That was $500 well spent. The new windshield wipers were swishing vigorously, giving me clear visibility and the brakes were firm.

I pressed speed dial where I had programmed them some time ago, and said, "Hello, it's me. Everything all right? I will be there in five minutes."

Hearing a not-so-calm woman's voice in the background, Meir answered, "I think we're getting close! What should I do?"

"Call an ambulance. I should arrive before them."

In a panic, worried that the ambulance may not make it, he'd forgotten the emergency number.

"It's 101. Call 101," I told him.

The rains after a dry spell made the roads more slippery than usual. At the first turn into the neighborhood where I was heading, I slowed down. At the next turn, the brakes were my friends as I pumped them. Making the last turn, I slowed down even more before arriving at their street, the steering wheel, veering to the right, seemed to be on a different system. The wheel was not turning to where I was directing the tires to go. *No, please G-d, no!* Straight ahead, flanking the sidewalk was an eight-foot-high stone wall surrounding an apartment complex. Coming up the road onto which I was trying to turn was a taxi driver.

Go faster. Or slow down! Just get out of my way!

At the rate he was traveling up from the right, I knew I

would plow straight into him. I said a short prayer and two seconds later everything went blank. The next thing I heard were voices saying, "Get out of the car. It could explode." Opening my lids slowly, I saw before me steam rising out from the hood of my car. I reached down to release myself from my seat belt.

In the black of night, the rain still misting down from the heavens, I held my arms outward toward two men, who pulled me from the car.

Lying on the cold wet ground, my teeth were chattering so hard I thought, *If these were dentures, they would have cracked and fallen out.*

"Where is the taxi driver?" I asked. "Is he okay?" Then I switched gears. "Go to building 102. A lady is giving birth. Go to 102. She is alone with her husband."

The ambulance wasn't here yet. The EMTs who volunteered in the area didn't believe me. "Please go to 102. A lady is having a baby there and they are alone."

No one believed me. Why should they? I forgot to mention that I was a doula on my way to a birth. They thought I was delirious from a concussion. Then their beepers went off. "A lady is having a baby in her house. Building 102." I was vindicated. Two EMTs headed off to the building with very little information. The two who stayed at my side until my ambulance came gave the two EMTs directions, with my help, on exactly how to enter the building. Five minutes later I asked, "What is happening? I am so cold, so cold."

A sympathetic person laid his jacket over my shivering body. The ambulance arrived to brace my neck and slide me onto a stretcher. The police report had been filled out in the interim. Name, identity number, and was I wearing a seat belt were the first three pieces of information requested.

They told me that mother and baby were fine. "She had the baby at home. All is well."

I smiled with delight. "*Mazel tov!* So, what was it?"

"A boy," one of the EMTs responded.

As they carried me away, I closed my eyes, thanking G-d I could speak and my arms and neck could move.

I was wheeled into a large, high-ceilinged room. I felt powerless as I was told not to move. My body was transferred from stretcher to X-ray table as they begin a series of ultrasounds with a machine wheeled next to my table. After hearing that my organs survived the trauma, the X-rays began. My swollen, throbbing foot was a big focus. Still waiting for a taxi to bring my husband to the hospital, a half-hour drive from our house, I tried to communicate to someone so I could have human, not only machine, contact. My Hebrew was fine — language was not the issue. They were focusing on their job, and right now I was a body to them and they were focusing on finding and fixing problems.

Finally, a lovely ultrasound technician told me, in a reassuring voice, that things looked very good. I asked her if she would like to work in the delivery ward. "I am a doula. Your pleasant smile and calm demeanor would be much appreciated there!"

As I was wheeled into the adjacent emergency room, I saw Moshe coming down the hall. "I am sorry, Moshe. I am so sorry..." I didn't know what made me feel worse — killing his night's sleep or crashing our car. We had canceled our comprehensive insurance for financial reasons. The obligatory insurance would cover only the taxi driver and personal liability.

Moshe, who never got in an accident in his life, said, "It's okay, it's okay." He is such a careful driver. He is so careful that I sometimes got annoyed at the lower-than-speed-limit pace he drove while allowing others to pass him. And now look — I had totaled the car. Moshe arrived at my side. Looking at me all he said was, "Are you okay?"

I responded, "I am so sorry. Really I am sorry."

We waited as the doctor came to give his assessment. "Your left foot is not broken."

Not broken? It is triple the normal size, lying sideways like a clubfoot, and very bruised. Holding back tears from the pain, I said, "Doctor, I have had sprains and torn ligaments in my life, but this is different. Please check again. It is really killing me."

He looked at me as if thinking, *Who is she to question me?* He pressed on the bottom of my heel, which was not at all in pain. "Okay," he said to my husband. "Take her back for two more X-rays." He scribbled something on a paper, handing it to Moshe. I was touring the hallways once again.

A few more clicks had us returning to the emergency department with the new X-rays. The man in white said, "I have good news and bad news for you."

"The bad news first, please."

"You have three small breaks," he reported. "But the good news is it looks like you won't need an operation."

I sighed a breath of relief, thinking, *He would have sent me home!* I am so glad I am a childbirth advocate. This is what I try to teach women, to think for themselves and speak up for what they feel their body wants and needs. I felt better as the warm plaster wound around my foot and leg to help me heal.

I called Suri, who was at another hospital in the labor and delivery unit. *"Mazel tov!"* I said to her husband, who answered the cell phone.

"I am sorry we couldn't wait for you," he replied.

"I understand. Do you know I was one minute away from your house when I crashed our car? I am in another hospital with three small breaks in my foot."

"Oh, no!" Meir exclaimed. "We had no idea what happened to you!"

"The EMTs probably didn't want to upset you, so they didn't tell you."

A day later, I called the taxi driver who informed me that he had badly bruised ribs but was okay. He was one of the two men who pulled me from the car. When he came to pick up insurance papers from our house a couple of days later, he said to my husband, "Be happy she is alive. I went to a kabbalist (mystic) living in Mea Shearim. He told me I was sent as an emissary to save her life. My car stopped your car from skidding into the stone wall. It was a true miracle." Chills travelled up and down my spine and arms. Now I was certain that the work I was doing was holy work.

In *The Ethics of the Fathers*, Rabbi Tarfun, a second century Jewish sage wrote: It is not incumbent upon you to finish the task. Yet, you are not free to desist from it.

Endnotes

IN THE EARLY 1960's ICEA (International Childbirth Education Association) and Lamaze were forerunners in childbirth education, followed in the 1980's, by ALACE (Association of Labor Assistants and Childbirth Educators) which incorporated doula training. In 1983 DONA (Doulas of North America), was the first established exclusively doula training organization. Now there are many: CAPPA (1998), Childbirth International (2000), followed by Hypno-Doula, Birthing from Within, Hypnobirthing, and many more in Australia and England. There are incredible women such as Paulina (Polly) Perez, working in the field of childbirth for over 40 years as a nurse, childbirth educator, doula trainer and author of the first book about doulas called *Special Women*.

Though these courses may emphasize different approaches how to offer support during the childbirth process, their goals were essentially the same—to empower women to have a positive, natural, meaningful birth.

From the various published studies, beginning with *The Doula Book* by Dr. Marshall and Phyllis Marshall Klaus(first published in1993) and the research of Dr. John Kennell and Dr. Ellen D. Hodnett, there is now strong evidence that corroborates what we suspected all along.

Doulas, by giving *continuous* physical and emotional support throughout the labor, result in increasing satisfaction for women in their birth experience.

Continuous support for women during childbirth
— Ellen D Hodnett[1,*], Simon Gates[2], G Justus Hofmeyr[3], Carol Sakala[4]

Twenty-two trials involving 15,288 women met inclusion criteria and provided usable outcome data. Results are of random-effects analyses, unless otherwise noted. Women allocated to continuous support were more likely to have a spontaneous vaginal birth (RR 1.08, 95% confidence interval (CI) 1.04 to 1.12) and less likely to have intrapartum analgesia (RR 0.90, 95% CI 0.84 to 0.96) or to report dissatisfaction (RR 0.69, 95% CI 0.59 to 0.79). In addition, their labors were shorter (MD -0.58 hours, 95% CI -0.85 to -0.31), they were less likely to have a caesarean (RR 0.78, 95% CI 0.67 to 0.91) or instrumental vaginal birth (fixed-effect, RR 0.90, 95% CI 0.85 to 0.96), regional analgesia (RR 0.93, 95% CI 0.88 to 0.99), or a baby with a low five-minute Apgar score (fixed-effect, RR 0.69, 95% CI 0.50 to 0.95).

There was no apparent impact on other intrapartum interventions, maternal or neonatal complications, or breastfeeding. Subgroup analyses suggested that continuous support was most effective when the provider was neither part of the hospital staff nor the woman's social network, and in settings in which epidural analgesia was not routinely available. No conclusions could be drawn about the timing of onset of continuous support. Also, due to fewer inductions and interventions, there are higher Apgar scores (evaluation of baby's breathing, muscle tone, etc.) and less admission to NICU (Neonatal Intensive Care Unit).

"If a Doula were a drug, it would be unethical not to use it."
—Dr. Marshall Klaus, MD, co-author of Mothering the Mother

About the Author

SARAH GOLDSTEIN IS a certified doula (15 years) and doula trainer for DONA (Doulas of North America) International (8 years). She is a natural childbirth advocate, promoting safer and more empowering birth experiences through organizing over a half-dozen seminars, creating CDs on pregnancy and childbirth for the Jewish woman, and writing articles for local and international magazines. She also has opened over 14 pregnancy and birth lending libraries.

Her first book, *Special Delivery*, was published by Targum Press in 2004. *More Special Deliveries* (2007) has chapter layouts by topics and more medical information.

Sarah has 6 children and 8 grandchildren (so far), most living in the Jerusalem area. She has merited attending their births, as well as 1400 others!

Contact Sarah at:
sardoula@gmail.com
http://jerusalemdoula.com
16/8 Astora Street
Jerusalem 97451, Israel

Printed in Great Britain
by Amazon